WOMEN AND AUTOIMMUNE DISEASE

WOMEN AND
AUTOIMMUNE
DISEASE

The Mysterious Ways Your Body Betrays Itself

MULTIPLE SCLEROSIS ★	FIBROMYALGIA
JUVENILE DIABETES ★	GRAVES' DISEASE
LUPUS ★	RHEUMATIC FEVER
CHRONIC FATIGUE SYNDROME ★	ANTIPHOSPHOLIPID SYNDROME
RHEUMATOID ARTHRITIS ★	PANDAS
SCLERODERMA ★	SJÖGREN'S SYNDROME
VASCULITIS ★	ALOPECIA

ROBERT G. LAHITA, M.D., Ph.D.

WITH INA YALOF

1❿ ReganBooks
Celebrating Ten Bestselling Years
An Imprint of HarperCollins*Publishers*

This book contains advice and information relating to health care. It is not intended to replace medical advice and should be used to supplement rather than replace regular care by your doctor. It is recommended that you seek your physician's advice before embarking on any medical program or treatment. All efforts have been made to assure the accuracy of the information contained in this book as of the date of publication. The publisher and the author disclaim liability for any medical outcomes that may occur as a result of applying the methods suggested in this book.

A hardcover edition of this book was published in 2004 by ReganBooks, an imprint of HarperCollins Publishers.

WOMEN AND AUTOIMMUNE DISEASE.
Copyright © 2004 by Robert G. Lahita.

FIRST PAPERBACK EDITION PUBLISHED 2005.

Designed by Pauline Neuwirth

The Library of Congress has cataloged the hardcover edition as follows:

Lahita, Robert G. (Robert George), 1945–
    Women and autoimmune disease : the mysterious ways your body betrays itself / Robert G. Lahita, with Ina Yalof.
        p.   cm.
    Includes index.
    ISBN 0-06-008149-X
    1. Women—Diseases.   2. Autoimmune diseases.   I. Yalof, Ina L., 1939– II. Title.

RG101.L33 2004
616.97'8'0082—dc22
                                                                    2004046775
ISBN 0-06-008150-3 (pbk.)

05 06 07 08 09 WBC/RRD 10 9 8 7 6 5 4 3 2

To George and Pauline

ACKNOWLEDGMENTS

I WOULD LIKE to recognize a number of people who have contributed in one way or another to this book. Let me begin chronologically. I am forever indebted to my publisher, Judith Regan, who made this book happen because she so strongly believed that all women should know about these illnesses. Special gratitude goes to my remarkably perceptive and sagacious editor, Cassie Jones, whose unending questions kept me on the right path and who shaped this manuscript to make it accessible to all readers. Pam Bernstein, my good friend and original agent, encouraged me to write this book, despite my claim that numerous other duties would never allow it. Thanks, too, to Barbara Lowenstein, my current agent for her dogged persistence and excellent representation. Both of these women had tremendous faith in the importance of this project and both connected me to Ina Yalof, a jewel in the world of writing, who made a dry manuscript sparkle and who guided this book to fruition.

Appreciation to Annie Krasnow for suggesting the title for this book and to my writer-son, Jason, who gave me many helpful comments. He, my son Eric, and my wife, Terry, encouraged me every step of the way.

Perhaps the most special acknowledgment goes to my patients with autoimmune diseases, many of whose stories I tell here, in one form or another. They continue to inspire me with their courage, perseverance, and expectation that tomorrow will be a new and better day.

CONTENTS

Contents

PART THREE: TREATMENTS

INTRODUCTION

⌒

AUTOIMMUNITY IS A biologic condition in which the immune system attacks the body it was created to protect. Autoimmune disorders are often repeatedly misdiagnosed because the symptoms are the only clue, and symptoms can be so variable. Consequently, patients can sometimes see four or five different medical specialists before they find one who can tell them what they have. No one knows what causes or triggers autoimmune disease and, again, there are many possibilities. For example, in one third of the cases there may be a family history, but in two thirds there is none. Researchers looking for causes still can only speculate on whether the environment—including anything from hair dye to hormones in food—infection, genetics, or a combination of these activate the autoimmune diseases, which affect millions of people worldwide.

I have written this book in an effort to make this complex topic as easy as possible for patients to understand. But it is meant to be relevant beyond the scope of just patients. It also is directed at families, friends, physicians, and anyone with an interest in autoimmune diseases, biology, and illness. The thrust of the book is toward women, because autoimmune diseases affect women far more often than they affect men. No one knows *why* this predilection exists, but it appears that just being a female, taking birth control pills, having a menstrual cycle, or getting pregnant can influence the immune system and accentuate or cause autoimmunity. The fact that most autoimmune diseases occur in women of childbearing age suggests that the sex hormones have a major influence. I have always held the theory that women must have more intricate immune systems than men because they are biologically equipped for pregnancy. Consider that a fetus—50 percent of which is as foreign as a transplanted organ—is carried for nine months without being rejected.

An equally important reason for this book's emphasis on women is that the autoimmune diseases are among the largest killers of young women in the world, and probably the greatest cause of women's disability. I believe it is absolutely essential that women understand as much as possible about these conditions, yet very few do. This continues to amaze me because, statistically, the incidence of autoimmune diseases rivals the far better known diseases. For example, in 1997 in America—the most recent data available at this time—autoimmune diseases affected some 5 to 8 percent of the population, or 14 to 22 million people. By comparison, in that same year, cancer affected 9 million people, and 22 million had heart disease.

So why, if the incidence of these diseases is so similar, are autoimmune diseases so rarely recognized? I have no answer. I only hope, indeed, I expect, that by the time you finish reading this book, you will be so well versed in the subject that you will be able to share your knowledge not only with your friends and family, but perhaps with your physician as well. We all love to learn something new.

Speaking for myself, I have always sought and revered *any* knowledge concerning the processes of life. When I first studied biology as a teenager, I was completely awestruck by everything that lived, from leaves to ants. I converted the family cellar into a small zoo and raised assorted creatures, from alligators to boa constrictors. A year later, when I was introduced to chemistry, the minizoo was out, and in came a laboratory full of wonderful things designed to excite a fifteen-year-old aspiring scientist. (Our neighbors were not quite as thrilled. It seems on several occasions a toxic gas I devised spewed forth from our cellar window through my jerry-rigged chemical-fume hood, killing their well-manicured lawn and shrubs.)

I came of age as a physician during the same years that science was laying the foundations for the study of autoimmunity, years that were marked by a progression of marvelous discoveries about the human body and new techniques to study the inner workings of cells. When I was in medical school in the 1960s, knowledge about the immune system was both limited and complicated. While scientists knew about many cells and tissues and how certain conditions manifested themselves, diseases such as multiple sclerosis and lupus still were not well characterized.

As I graduated from medical school and began my training in internal medicine at Cornell Medical College, antibodies and toxic cells were just being discovered, and because this new research fascinated me, in my final year of residency I took a three-week elective in immunology. I was fortunate to have my choice of key scientists with whom to study for those weeks. I chose Professor Henry G. Kunkel, the immunology genius of Rockefeller University, not only for his stellar reputation, but also because I had longed to work at Rockefeller ever since Sinclair Lewis profiled it in the book *Arrowsmith*, and because it is considered to be a Nobel laureate factory.

Rockefeller turned out to be everything I had hoped it would be. Most of the grandfathers of the science of immunology came through our laboratories, and I had the wonderful good fortune to work alongside many of them as they established the concepts that formed the basis for much of what we now know about autoimmune diseases. But it was Dr. Kunkel who was the prize. During those early weeks he became my mentor, and he was the reason I remained at Rockefeller for the next eleven years, starting with a Fellowship, evolving as a researcher, and finally becoming a professor in the field of immunology and clinical research.

Today, thirty years later, according to the American Autoimmune Related Disease Association, there may be as many as eighty known autoimmune diseases—and probably many more in which autoimmunity is the real but unconfirmed cause. (More on what defines an autoimmune disease in the following two chapters.) I must say, it has been an extraordinary experience for me to have grown up in medicine while my field of interest has developed and matured as well.

In this book, I hope to illuminate the many facets of autoimmune disease, including the ways it affects human behavior and everyday life, the difficulties involved in getting a solid and timely diagnosis from the medical community, and the very latest and most cutting-edge ideas and treatments for these mysterious illnesses. In Part I, the first chapter lays the groundwork by describing the normal immune system and how it works. Chapter 2 is an overview of autoimmune diseases in general. What we do not know, as I mentioned earlier, is precisely *why* the body begins to attack itself—but there is much that we do know, and here I describe the process of autoimmunity as well as the most current information on the mechanisms and various theories behind the *diseases* as a whole.

The essence of the book is found in Part II, which includes fifteen chapters that deal with specific diseases. But before going further, I would like to note two important things: First, the cases that are presented in each of the examples of particular diseases are, in many situations, amalgams of actual cases. But while I have changed the names and circumstantial details to protect the patients, I have made every effort to preserve the salient details of their diseases and the essential experiences and feelings of the women themselves. Second, there are so many different autoimmune diseases that it clearly is impossible to portray all of them, if only because of space constraints. So, I have selected fifteen. The process of selection, while a writer's prerogative, is also the writer's responsibility. I have tried to be both representational and evenhanded with my selections. For example, I have tried to include the common and the less common diseases, the organ specific and the systemic, those that afflict adults and those that strike only children, and so on. Many readers will look for their disease here and not find it. I regret that I have left out so many, but in fact, the information included in each of these disease-specific chapters is in many ways relevant to all autoimmune diseases. As you read them, they will clearly enhance your understanding of autoimmune diseases as a whole.

Most autoimmune diseases overlap in one way or another, and many people, as you will see, suffer from more than one. For the purpose of continuity, I have attempted to group the diseases as sequentially as possible. For example, chapter 3 describes *antiphospholipid (sticky blood) syndrome* and is followed in chapter 4 by *idiopathic thrombocytopenic purpura (ITP),* because both diseases involve the blood and platelets. *Juvenile diabetes, PANDAS,* and *rheumatic fever* are next, and these strike mostly children and young adults. While juvenile diabetes involves antibodies against the insulin receptors on the cells depriving them of food for energy, PANDAS and rheumatic fever in part are affected by the brain's wiring. *Multiple sclerosis,* which can take up to two years to diagnose, also affects the brain, as does *vasculitis,* a disease of the blood vessels that can become critical in a matter of minutes.

Lupus, the next chapter, is considered the great mimic of other diseases and has symptoms too numerous to mention here. One of them, however, can be hair loss, which is the subject of the chapter on *alopecia universalis,* a disease in which women can permanently lose all their body hair. While they may feel perfectly well, these women suffer the symptoms of their disease in other ways. *Sjögren's syndrome,* in which antibodies attack the tear and saliva glands, rendering them almost useless, affects more people that one might expect, considering how few have heard of it. One of my patients with Sjögren's described it best when she said, "Even if I wanted to cry about this, I couldn't."

Autoimmune *thyroid disease* is quite common, particularly *Graves' disease,* which made its media debut several years ago when George Bush and his wife, Barbara, developed the disease while in the White House. *Autoimmune liver disease,* which follows in the next chapter, is far more rare than Graves' disease, but also more deadly. Fortunately, it is correctable if caught early; the patient described in this chapter is now the recipient of a liver transplant and was last seen (by me) riding a horse in Central Park. *Scleroderma* is a disease that is easy to diagnose and hard to treat. Conversely, as you will see when you meet Vicki, the ballerina, *polymyositis* is hard to diagnose, but once you make the diagnosis, it is easy to treat. *Rheumatoid arthritis* is the most common autoimmune disease and, at the same time, the one that offers the most hope. I have two patients who could hardly walk when I met them and who now run marathons. Considering what we knew twenty-five years ago about how to diagnose and treat autoimmune diseases, I believe this is nothing short of miraculous.

The last chapter covers *chronic fatigue syndrome* and *fibromyalgia,* two of what I consider the mystery diseases—that is, syndromes that might be autoimmune but as yet have no defined autoimmune mechanisms. But these diseases are so inextricably linked to so many autoimmune illnesses that I have chosen to give them a place in this book. Issues that are more controversial surround the *silicone breast implant syndromes,* which have autoimmune characteristics and are thought by many to be the perfect examples of environmentally produced autoimmunity. I am not sure I agree, but I have presented the issue as fairly as I know how.

The final two chapters deal with the very latest treatments for the symptoms of autoimmune diseases: drugs and alternative and complementary therapies. The goal for autoimmune disease is to develop drugs that control the overactive immune system without killing its functions and ultimately causing infection or even death. The chapter on drugs explores the latest pharmaceuticals to help the reader understand how and why the new treatments work. The chapter on alternative and complementary therapies includes the homeopathic regimes and nonpharmacological means of treating autoimmunity.

Women and Autoimmune Disease contains a great deal of new information. In the last thirty years, more advances have been made in the area of immunology than in any other area of medicine. We can thank the molecular biologists for this. However, even they have benefited from Mother Nature's munificence—they use the many antibodies described in this book to study the fundamentals of cell function and the processes of living. I am hopeful that we will see a continued exponential rise of medical advances in this area in the near future. For now, however, I feel strongly that every day of life in the future for the autoimmune patient can realistically be lived with the hope that "today is the day they will understand my illness." Indeed, I expect to see the time when the cases of the patients in this book are nothing more than historical curiosities.

PART ONE

What Is an Autoimmune Disease?

CHAPTER ONE

THE IMMUNE SYSTEM

First Line of Defense

OR MOST OF us who go about the everyday tasks of work, shopping, or life in general, the immune system does not seem particularly remarkable. Why would it be? Few movies of the week have been made about it. There are no weekend telethons on its behalf. It does not have a star such as Britney Spears anxious to attach her name to it, nor does Katie Couric remind us to have it checked every year, or two, or five.

No, it is just there, doing its job of protecting us from the, oh, say 5 or 6 billion molecules of viruses, bacteria, parasites, pollutants, and germs to which we open our doors—not to mention our mouths—every single day of our lives. When things are going smoothly, we are all a bit guilty of a laissez-faire attitude about the immune system. Ah, but let something go awry and watch out! *Now* it has our attention.

And well it should.

We cannot live, at least not very well, without our immune systems. The immune system is the body's natural defense mechanism against the attackers I have cited above—as well as many as-yet-unknown microbes that would love nothing more than to climb inside and set up shop all over our bodies. To get a good sense of the might of this silent but hardworking system, consider what happens to something living once it dies: Within minutes, everything shuts down; within hours the process of decomposition sets in, and long before sunset, the body is completely taken over by all sorts of unwelcome visitors. I need not go further. You get the picture.

If you are in any way concerned about autoimmune disease—and I suspect you are if you're reading this book—it is essential that you understand the basic workings of the *healthy* immune system. This chapter explains it, but be forewarned; in large part, it will be a vocabulary lesson. Many of the terms I use here are repeated throughout the book, so it is helpful to understand them from the first. I do promise this, however: To the extent that it is possible to illustrate things clearly otherwise, I will not burden you with so much as an extraneous microbe.

How Does the Immune System Work?

Central to the workings of the immune system is its ability to distinguish between what is "us" and what is "not us," hereafter known as *self* and *nonself*. Every cell in the body carries distinctive molecules that distinguish it as "self." When foreign—"nonself"—molecules enter the body, if they trigger an immune reaction, they are known as *antigens* (against self).

Antigens can come from outside the body or may actually exist as part of the body itself. An external antigen could be a bacterium, a virus, or a parasite, for example. Tissues or cells from other humans, such as those introduced during a heart or lung transplant, also are recognized as antigens, which is why, without strong drugs to suppress the immune system, the body rejects transplanted organs. As soon as the immune system recognizes an antigen in the bloodstream, it responds by producing *antibodies*, which are molecules designed to counteract the antigen and render it impotent. The process of creating an antibody upon recognition of an antigen is known as an *immune response*.

For an example of an internal antigen, there are times when the immune system suddenly turns on the hair follicles, mistakenly recognizing them as foreign and makes antibodies against them. This constitutes an *autoimmune response* that can result in an autoimmune disease called *alopecia areata universalis,* or complete loss of hair. The hair follicle itself has become the antigen and is now called an *autoantigen.* Why cells in the body that heretofore coexisted in peace suddenly become the enemy, no one knows.

Organs of the Immune System

The organs that comprise the immune system include the bone marrow, the lymph nodes, the thymus, and the spleen. These organs are connected to each other and to other organs of the body by way of the lymphatic vessels, a network that courses throughout the body in a manner similar to the blood vessels.

The *bone marrow* serves as the factory that produces, among other things, the white blood cell (also known as *leukocytes*) a collection of different kinds of cells, such as polymorphonuclear leukocytes (phagocytes), monocytes, and lymphocytes. They are considered the backbone of the immune system, and many of them are described below.

The *lymph nodes* are small bean-shaped structures that contain filter tissue and work as the clearinghouse for germs and foreign invaders. They are the place where the immune cells face off with antigens. Using a police force as an analogy for the immune system, you might consider the lymph nodes as police precincts that are strategically placed in various parts of the body where the immune system has to be on high alert—for example, the tonsils, the ears, the mouth, the genitals, or any area where there might be an invasion of a foreign substance or a foreign germ. When fighting a bacterial infection, for example, the nodes are the battleground for bacteria and the immune cells that are fighting them. The result of this influx of cells and cell activity is a swollen lymph node, which is a good predictor that an infection exists.

The *thymus,* which is located in the middle of the chest under the breastbone and below the thyroid gland, is the master programmer of the immune system. Interestingly, the thymus usually disappears by the time a person is twenty-five, once its workings are well in place. This disappearance of the thymus, through a process called programmed cell death, is one of the most studied phenomena in cell biology, because no one knows what causes it. We know only that the thymus gland shrinks and ultimately disappears with the aid of male hormones called *androgens*.

The *spleen*, the least important organ of the four, is the dumping site for cellular garbage, including foreign matter picked up by the immune system's scavenger cells. In the spleen, the refuse is digested into the smallest of molecular parts, which are then recycled as innocuous substances.

Cells of the Immune System

The most important of the immune cells are the white blood cells, which have many varieties. Among the most prominent and hardest working are the *lymphocytes*, the cells that have receptors for antigens on their surface. They are comprised of two major categories— *T cells* and *B cells*. Still other lymphocytes become natural killer cells that attack tumor cells. Most lymphocytes have different assignments, all of which, together, focus on keeping us protected.

▷ *T Cells*

As they travel throughout the body on the lookout for foreign invaders, T cells provide help to the immune defenses in two ways. Some regulate the operations of the immune system, while others are poisonous and strike out at antigens directly to demolish them. When a T cell detects a foreign invader, it immediately orchestrates a manifold response. That response includes stimulating the B cells to secrete antibodies and calling other T cells into action. T cells are the ones largely responsible for the rejection of tissue grafts and transplanted organs.

How does a T cell recognize an antigen? On the surface of each cell is a package of molecules called a *major histocompatibility complex* (MHC), also known as the *human leukocyte antigen* (HLA). The MHC sits on the cell membrane and recognizes what is and is not self. On recognition of an enemy in its midst, the MHC marks the antigen so that the T cells can recognize it. When they do, the T cells issue orders for other cells to manufacture *cytokines* and *chemokines,* the chemicals that help to destroy the invaders.

I should point out that every cell has many receptors on its surface that recognize a variety of things, from hormones to antigens. The immune system, in all of its wisdom, will not allow a single receptor to make an immune response. It requires a number of receptors working in unison. The MHC is only one such receptor. The requirement for multiple receptors acting to recognize an antigen establishes a failsafe mechanism for normal immune function. It is similar to what would happen if the president of the United States had a locked box that contained a button that could send a missile halfway across the world. In order to launch the missile, the president would have to have a key, but so would the secretary of state and the vice president. For the most part, the immune system has this same kind of built-in safeguard so that the wrong tissues are not rejected.

▷ Cytokines and Chemokines

Cytokines are considered the working tools of T cells. Cytokines are molecules that are responsible for intercellular communication within the immune system as well as for information interchange between the immune system and other systems of the body. Because they also carry messages between cells, I refer to them as "communication molecules." Cytokines direct cellular traffic and help destroy target cells—including cancer cells—by attaching themselves to the specific receptors on the target cells.

While the cytokines do good work for the immune system, they can produce adverse effects as well, such as fever, malaise, pain, and wasting. But these side effects are simply part of getting the job done. For example, it is thought that fever comes because the cytokines have an impact on the temperature-regulating mechanism in the brain.

Chemokines are small molecules that, like cytokines, in their efforts to do good can become overzealous and eventually cause trouble. For example, overproduction of certain chemokines in the joints of people with rheumatoid arthritis may eventually result in a destructive invasion of the joint space. The inflammation is what causes the redness, swelling, and pain in so many of the autoimmune diseases.

▷ *B Cells*

While T cells appear to run the show, B cells are equally useful in their supporting role. The chief job of B cells is to mature into *plasma cells*. Each plasma cell makes specific antibodies that seek and destroy specific foreign antigens. When a B cell locates an antigen, it binds itself to the antigen and labels it for destruction. A B cell can make antibodies when told to do so by a T cell, and sometimes it can act on its own accord.

▷ *Macrophages and Neutrophils*

These are additional weapons used by the immune system. They are neither B nor T cells, but rather separate types of white blood cells that have their own specific functions. The macrophage circulates in the blood, and when it finds an antigen it attaches to it and presents it to the MHC, which, as we have just seen, gets the immune response going. When the antigen is demolished, the leftover debris is then carried by the neutrophils to the spleen and eventually excreted from the body.

This may be more than you ever wanted to know, but I am guessing that by now you have a healthy respect for the immune system. As you can see, it requires an exquisitely delicate balance to keep the system performing at top function but still reigned in—that is, to keep it running without running amok.

Immune Memory

To me, the most fascinating thing about the entire immune system is that it remembers. It is the only organ in the body, other than the brain, that has memory. Even now, in middle age, my immune system can recognize foreign substances that I was exposed to back in nursery school. (So can yours.) It is why, after I caught chickenpox at age seven, I never got it again, even when my own children brought it into our house. Considering the millions of antigens that it is possible to be exposed to, this is quite a remarkable feat. However, since the brain is capable of recalling all sorts of things from childhood, some we even wish we could forget, it should not surprise us that the immune system can conjure up memories as well.

The doors to the memory bank open whenever T cells and B cells are activated in the face of antigens. At that point, some portion of those cells become "memory" cells, so when a person encounters that same antigen again, the immune system is primed to destroy it quickly. In other words, exposure to an antigen early in life (in this case, through inactivated infectious agents) usually provides what we call *long-term immunity*, or protection throughout life. This is the theory behind vaccination. A vaccination is an injection of a tiny amount of the germ—small enough not to be dangerous—that provokes your own immune system to make antibodies against it. Because the immune system has a long memory, when the antigen again reappears, the antibodies will be resynthesized as a response. In this way, you are protected for the rest of your life. This is why, as we mentioned above, people rarely get chickenpox more than once.

Short-term immunity can be conferred as well, but rather than for use as a long-term protective measure like vaccination, this medical treatment is short-lived and reserved for more acute situations. For example, if you get a snake bite, you will be given an antitoxin, that is, an antibody-containing serum that has been created in the laboratory from antibodies of humans or animals. If you step on a rusty nail, you most certainly will be given a tetanus shot, which is essentially tetanus antitoxin. These antitoxins work for a set amount of time and eventually leave the body. Similarly, antibodies from their mothers, as we well know, protect infants, both before birth and through the first few months of life.

Women and Immunity: The Influence of Gender on the Immune System

Why is there such a seemingly unfair preponderance of women associated with practically every one of the autoimmune diseases? In addition to the microbes that cunningly sneak past what we think are impenetrable barriers (the skin, for example) to break into our bodies, certain other influences also can directly or indirectly affect the workings of the immune system. As it turns out, one of the greatest factors that influence the immune system is gender.

I have a theory (although it is not scientifically proven yet) that women are so prone to autoimmune disease because by nature their immune systems are so much more complicated and finely tuned than men's. (You know what happens to complex machinery. Consider a dishwasher with twenty-two buttons as opposed to one with a simple on/off button. Which machine is the first to break?)

A woman must be prepared to carry, for nine months, a fetus that is 50 percent antigenic (nonself). Think about it. Half of the genes in a baby belong to the father, a total stranger to a woman's body, and yet the unborn child is never rejected by her immune system. To the contrary, her immune system has the wisdom to turn parts of itself off for those nine months and instead treat her developing baby like one of the family. It does this through many mechanisms, one of which is called a *blocking complex,* which impedes the recognition of a foreign antigen in the body, but only in the fetus, not in the rest of the body. During pregnancy, hormonal and immune functions operate at their highest level and, as you will see when we discuss the individual diseases, the immune system takes on an unusual character. Some say that it is weakened while others suggest that it is strengthened. I believe it is a little bit of both; the immune system is strengthened in the mother herself and weakened when it comes to the fetus, the placenta, and the uterus. How it knows is another one of the miracles of nature and science that keep me in awe.

Other Influences on the Immune System

▷ *Disease*

Certain diseases can weaken or kill the immune system. Viruses can infect a variety of different cells and be very damaging to the immune system, particularly when they choose to infect T cells or B cells selectively. Hepatitis B and hepatitis C are known to weaken the immune system. The HIV virus does, too. In fact, this virus is a master at infecting the "T helper" cells, also known as CD4 cells. As the infection progresses, the CD4 type of T cells begin to disappear and the patient's immune system becomes increasingly deficient. Other types of infections that take advantage of a weakened immune system include the herpesvirus (fever blisters or shingles, which appear during times of stress), pneumonia, and meningitis. I have seen everything from bone marrow failure to arthritis develop in response to viruses in a person with a compromised immune system.

▷ Stress

The immune system—like the brain—can be affected by brain chemicals such as endorphins. We know from the scientific literature that such internal opiates are quite powerful and affect not only the way we think but also the way we handle foreign invaders. Many years ago, scientists investigated the effects of synthetic endorphins on immune function in animals and were surprised at how dramatic they were. We learned that cell function and antibody secretion increase or decrease in the presence or absence of certain endorphins, and that cytokine production is increased in the presence of certain endorphins in a disease such as lupus. We do not know enough yet about the benefits of using drugs that suppress naturally existing opiates in patients with autoimmune disease, but I believe that this is a viable idea and hope that someone will one day seek funding for such a project.

▷ Genetics

We have long known that many diseases, such as sickle cell disease, cystic fibrosis, Huntington's disease, and Cooley's anemia, are passed down genetically from one relative to another. We know, too, that genetics plays a large role in how a person's immune system behaves—a role that extends to the success or failure of organ transplantation in an individual. To see if a transplanted organ will "take" and not be rejected by the immune system, we always look for a gene match on *chromosome 6*, which is the site of the immune response genes. These genes can make you susceptible to infection or can protect you from it. Immune response genes also are responsible for *immunodeficiency*, a rare condition in which the immune system is seriously compromised. This situation existed in the "bubble boy," a child named David Vetter, who spent much of his too-short life (1972–1984) in an airtight suit to ensure that no foreign matter entered his world. There is a certain risk imparted by the genes on chromosome 6, but having those genes or not having them does not guarantee that we will or will not get a particular autoimmune disease. This is discussed further in the following chapters.

▷ *Age*

I believe that as we get older, the immune system becomes less efficient, which is hardly surprising, since everything else in our bodies gets a bit worn around the edges as well. The late Lewis Thomas, a brilliant biologist, physician, and award-winning medical writer, put forth the idea of a loss of immune surveillance as the main mechanism for the development of cancer, not only in the aged but in the general population. I could not agree more. An age-induced decrease in immune surveillance cannot help but allow infections and perhaps cancers to more easily slip past the immune system's police force. We can probably avoid this somewhat by taking good care of ourselves as we get older. Of course, it is never too soon, or too late, to start.

▷ *Lifestyle Choices*

It is no secret that we can compromise our own immune systems in the choices we make in our lifestyles. Although it has not yet been scientifically proven, I strongly suspect that smoking affects the immune system. If this turns out to be so, then it could provide yet one more link in the smoking–cancer connection. Drinking most certainly has an affect on immune function. Chronic alcoholics are unceasingly immunosuppressed, which leaves them susceptible to infection. When a chronic alcoholic with a fever comes into the emergency room, the chances are very good that he or she has some infection that is going to be tough to treat. That is in part because alcohol compromises the ability of the neutrophils to pick up and carry away the garbage of the immune reaction. Those cells are paralyzed by drink, much like the person in whom they live. How much alcohol is too much is truly anyone's guess, however. As yet, there are no specific data to tell us.

Keeping the Immune System Healthy

Just as we can compromise our own immune system, we also can enhance it. Like the brain, the immune system must stay active and healthy in order to prevent it from aging before the rest of the body. The object is to keep it active without putting it to work defending against disease.

How do you keep an immune system active and healthy? Simple—by living well. By now, you know what that entails: eating a healthful diet, getting enough sleep, exercising, drinking only in moderation, and not overstressing yourself. But there are other important methods to be considered. For example:

▷ Avoid or, better still, prevent exposure to environmental toxins such as poisons, mercury, and heavy metals.

▷ Avoid taking any unnecessary drugs. Every drug we take as a medication has a trade-off, and some of it is probably detrimental to the immune function. For example, drugs such as Tagamet, which protects the lining of the stomach, also have an effect on the chemicals in the liver, which has to eventually clear the drugs from the body.

▷ Understand that diet can influence your immune system—and choose your foods wisely. Dietary influences and their effects on the immune system are currently being studied, but much is already known. For example, we know that consuming excessive hormones can affect the immune system in a very subtle way. Many of the cows, pigs, chickens, and turkeys we eat are fed hormones, and eating them may be tantamount to consuming hormones. But there are hormones in plants as well, so even a vegetarian is not necessarily free of hormones. Phytoestrogens—plant hormones—can affect the immune system in very subtle ways. Just eating a yam or a sweet potato may cause hormones to increase immune function. It is thought that estrogens boost the immune system, which is why women with autoimmune disease, whose immune systems are running rampant, should not be taking estrogen. Androgens (male hormones) have both a stimulatory and an inhibitory effect. One of the early theories linking gender and the immune system is that men do not have autoimmune disease in as great numbers as women because the androgens keep their immune systems in check.

▷ Have sex. Sexual activity is very good for immune function because it activates the hormones that are changed and regulated by the sex act. When a male has sex, his androgen levels rise. A woman's estrogen levels rise when she has sex, and she secretes androgens, although no one yet knows which hormone provides the benefit. As far as I am concerned, it is a very appropriate balance. In short: Sex is good for everyone. (I might add, however, that as far as I know, sex has no effect, one way or the other, on autoimmunity.)

An Example of a Normal Immune Response

Now that I have dissected the immune system into its many component parts, I want to reassemble it with an example that illustrates just how the normal immune system works. I have selected as my model a patient named Florence, whom I saw for the first time this morning as I made rounds in the hospital with the attending physicians, house staff, and students connected to the Department of Medicine. As is customary on rounds, medical students present patients at the bedside. During "presentation," the student, who has earlier evaluated the patient, leads the discussion of her case in front of the assembled physicians.

The first time is a rite of passage that every medical student goes through. This morning, a very apprehensive third-year medical student named Anne presented Florence to our group. Anne, just one week into her clinical rotations, was an incredibly young-looking woman (the students are getting younger every year) with dark curly hair. Her trembling voice as she spoke and the subtly nervous flutter of the hand in which she held her note cards belied her composed and self-assured facade.

While Florence's disease may not be very memorable, I can say with authority that Anne will never forget her, because I still remember when *I* was a third-year medical student presenting my first patient on rounds. I recall feeling utterly small that morning among the dozen or so white-coated physicians whom I followed, protocol style, into the hospital room and who ultimately surrounded the patient's bed like a picket fence. My patient was a frail, elderly woman, selected because she had a persistent high fever of unknown origin. Without once looking up from my note cards, I very nervously gave my presentation, describing her vital signs and the results of my earlier examination. Several minutes later, when I finished my presentation and was just about to breathe a sigh of relief, the chief of medicine started firing a torrent of questions at me, the answers to which I could not possibly have known. (It is an awful experience, known at some medical schools as "pipping the student," but at one point or another, all medical students seem to go through it.) I do know that by the time the ordeal was over, I was shaking as much if not more than the patient in the bed. I vowed then never to treat a student in that manner, and I do not believe I ever have.

This morning's presenter, Anne, reading from note cards, told us that Florence is a thirty-five-year-old accountant and the mother of three children all under twelve. She also volunteers as a reading assistant several hours a week at her daughter's school. This small bit of social history was important, if not essential, to know, because it helps the physician determine where an infection might have begun. Florence probably contracted her infection from her daughters or one of the children at the school, although we may never know for sure. Sometimes infections that slide unnoticed through populations of young children with resilient immune systems can provide a source of far more serious disease in adults, usually in people who have not been vaccinated for a particular illness or who have no immunity acquired naturally from previous infection.

Florence began feeling cold and clammy at work and decided to come home early and go to bed. She had a fever of 100 degrees by the time she got home, and by nighttime, the fever had spiked to 103 degrees. She spent a sleepless night with intermittent bouts of nausea and vomiting, which led her and her husband, Jack, to assume this was most likely stomach flu or some mild case of food poisoning, and that she would be better in twenty-four hours.

Although her fever dropped, she remained at home and in bed the following day. That evening, she experienced sharp chest pain that occasionally radiated to her neck. Moreover, her fever rose again to 103 degrees and was now accompanied by chills and extreme shaking. When no amount of blankets would keep his wife warm, and her chest pain started to worsen, Jack called 911. She was admitted to the hospital that evening.

From my perspective, it was clear that Florence had a plain, garden-variety bacterial infection. Her chest pain and the violent fever were simply the result of her body's attempt to get rid of it. The fever was caused by the body's secretion of certain cytokines that, as we saw earlier, can cause high fevers. Her chest pain was the result of the immune system confronting the bacteria in the lung, and leaving all sorts of wreckage in its wake.

Let us look again at what happens as the immune system goes to work: Florence is invaded by a bacterial infection she contracted from a child. As the bacteria enters the body, the antigen presenting cells—the macrophages that have been floating around the bloodstream patrolling for foreigners—recognize the bacteria as an antigen and immediately transmit this information to the T cells. The T cells secrete cytokines and chemokines, which in turn call for more T cells to come to the site of the injury. As these other cells come in, cytokines are released in great amounts, which causes the fever. Then the neutrophils come in to scoop up the damaged cells as well as most of the bacteria that are multiplying faster than the new cells are arriving. This leads to a collection of pus in the lung, which causes pain, swelling, redness, high fever, and inflammation.

What in fact was going on was a major pitched battle by her immune system to save Florence's lung. Using the full powers of the immune system, Florence's body was taking orders from her T and B cells and fighting back. Had it not, the bacteria would rapidly have taken over most of Florence's lung and invaded her bloodstream. It is anyone's guess where they might have ended up next had they not been stopped cold in her chest. In the very old and the very young, the bacteria might win. In those who do not have functioning immune systems, such as people with AIDS or whose immune systems are weakened by chemotherapy, the bacteria might also win. However, Florence was young and had been healthy. She was given IV antibiotics and was quickly on her way to recovery.

Florence is a classic example of a routine infection in a young woman whose normal immune system is simply doing its job. Conversely, autoimmune disease is the example of that same immune system in total disarray, the outcome of which can lead to combat on a far greater scale. Fighting the ravages of autoimmune disease is no small battle. Rather, as we shall see in the next chapter, it often can be all-out war.

CHAPTER TWO

AUTOIMMUNE DISEASES

AUTOIMMUNE DISEASE: A condition in which the process of autoimmunity, which is natural in small doses, goes out of control and results in rejection of specific parts within the body, as though all or some of those parts come from an unrelated individual.

*J*N CHAPTER 1, we saw how the immune system creates antibodies to defend the body against the onslaught of invading antigens—viruses, bacteria, or parasites. But sometimes an antigen so closely resembles healthy self-tissue (a situation called *mimicry*) that when the immune system unleashes antibodies against the foreign cells, they mistakenly attack and destroy good cells as well. These confused antibodies, known as *autoantibodies* because they turn against "self-tissue," are the cause of many adverse conditions that fall under the umbrella heading of *autoimmune diseases*. It never ceases to amaze me that such a full-blown field as autoimmunity, affecting tens of millions of people in this country, can be reduced to so simple a concept as an antibody or cell gone awry. But there it is.

I would like to insert a caveat here. As you read this book, you will notice that I often make the statement "we just don't know why" or "we're not quite sure." I am sorry we do not have all the answers, but scientifically speaking, this specialty is very young. Compared to much of the world of medicine, the field of autoimmunity is still in the embryonic stages.

The first historical mention of autoimmunity goes back in our recent history to the German biologist and pathologist Paul Ehrlich, who won the Nobel Prize for Medicine in 1908. Around the turn of the last century, Ehrlich coined the term *horror autotoxicus* (fear of self-poisoning) as the phenomenon that could occur when a person's own defenses turned against him or her. At the time, horror autotoxicus was largely a clinical observation about findings made in certain patients. Ehrlich was much involved in describing antigens and their chemical structure and looking at something new called *antitoxins*. He realized that an antigen, in addition to being foreign matter, also could be a part of our own tissues but would be perceived as foreign by the immune system. In short, he put forth the now-well-accepted theory that in addition to seeking out strangers, our immune systems can react to something that is native to our bodies. He did not know how or with what.

Around the same time, the great internist William Osler, a contemporary of Ehrlich, studied skin diseases that he thought were related to tuberculosis (TB), but actually were autoimmune diseases. Although he eventually concluded that these diseases were unique and not TB, he did not have the tools to prove their biological origins. It would be another fifty years until the immune system was defined and Ehrlich and Osler's observations were substantiated. Antibodies were not identified until the 1950s, so all these investigators dreamed creatively about what "might be," which is much the same process that all medical researchers use today.

A decade later, in the sixties, the concept of autoimmunity as a cause of human illness became part of the medical lore when doctors Gerald Edelman of Rockefeller University and Rodney Peters at Oxford University defined the structure of an antibody. This resulted in the development of laboratory tests to help recognize autoimmune diseases. Soon after, T cells and B cells were identified, and the discovery of the origins of antibodies and autoreactive cells made autoimmunity an active field of research in science and medicine. Considering that all of this happened in the last forty years, we have made astonishing progress.

The man who brought me into this field was the late Professor

Henry G. Kunkel of Rockefeller University. Dr. Kunkel, who died in 1983, made many seminal discoveries in his lifetime and changed science in so many ways. He was a laconic introvert who believed in the sanctity of the written word. He would never allow props such as slides or pictures to be used during a talk. Instead, we had a blackboard and were required to write out everything we considered important enough to share with our fellow students and professor. Most people outside of his laboratory thought him a curmudgeon, but to those who knew him well, he was a delightful person who had quite a sense of humor. For example, I trained with another graduate student from China who continually confused the words "sera" (plural) and "serum" (singular). Because Dr. Kunkel was such a stickler for scientific detail, he decided to teach her which was which, once and for all. One morning, he brought in a cowbell to the lecture hall and every time the student made that particular mistake, he would ring the bell. It drove this poor woman to distraction, but she quickly learned the difference. She is now a Ph.D. and the president of a very successful, large immunologic biotech company.

Dr. Kunkel inspired us all by using the simplest techniques to make the most remarkable discoveries. He pioneered the principle of using simplicity to explain complex phenomena, concluding that if you could show something in one human being, it was enough to prove a point. He and his students (he trained Gerald Edelman in the early 1960s) discovered and classified most of the autoantibodies we know today. But perhaps the most important contribution that he made to medicine was that he personally trained more autoimmune disease specialists than anyone else in history.

Defining Autoimmune Disease

Henry Kunkel would have been the first to agree that defining autoimmune disease does not come easily. At last count, there were more than eighty different autoimmune diseases, each of which acts upon the body in a different way. Sometimes a single organ is selected for attack, such as when the autoimmune reaction is directed against the brain in multiple sclerosis or the intestines in Crohn's disease. Other times, multiple organs become targets, which is called *systemic* autoimmune disease. Sometimes the cells are the targets, such as in systemic lupus erythematosus (SLE), polymyositis, and scleroderma. There are periods when a disease such as rheumatoid arthritis renders a patient only slightly achy, and other times when major flareups temporarily cripple her.

An autoimmune reaction can target any organ in the body. For example, the makeup of a certain strain of strep bacteria so closely mimics the tissues of the mitral valve of the heart that when the antibodies go after the strep bacteria, they unwittingly attack the heart tissue as well, which can lead to a disease called rheumatic fever. Then again, one disease can affect many organs or a single organ in more than one way. Consider that in Hashimoto's thyroiditis the immune system sets its sights on the thyroid gland, disrupting its functioning and ultimately causing secretion of very little thyroid hormone. With Graves' disease, on the other hand, the thyroid gland secretes excessive amounts of hormone.

Diagnosing Autoimmune Diseases

If it seems that these diseases are hard to define, they are even harder to diagnose—as anyone who has an autoimmune disease can testify. They are among the most poorly understood and recognized illnesses, which is why for so many patients it can and often does take years—even decades—to receive a correct diagnosis of a specific autoimmune disease.

Why are they so hard to diagnose? Let me give you an example. For most nonautoimmune diseases, a typical scenario is as follows: The doctor takes the patient's history, examines the patient, does some laboratory tests and perhaps some noninvasive studies, combines and evaluates the information, and makes the diagnosis. With autoimmune diseases, it is not nearly that easy, as you will see throughout the following chapters. We do take a history and perform a physical examination, but then the problems begin.

The main reason autoimmune disease is so difficult to diagnose is that there are no definitive diagnostic laboratory tests. Yes, we can produce antibodies in a blood test on a patient with suspected autoimmune disease, and we may even turn up an autoantibody. But the presence of an antibody only suggests that the patient has the disease. It is not specific; that is, it does not guarantee that the patient has the disease. The presence of autoreactive T cells or B cells are not specific, either, because healthy people sometimes have them too. So in cases where autoimmune disease is suspected, the laboratory tests merely support what the physician already suspects. What really creates the diagnosis is the clinical training and the clinical impression of the doctor, which is why it is so very important to find a well-trained specialist.

Beyond the clinical quandaries, there are many other situations that add to the difficulty of diagnosing autoimmune disease:

▷ Symptoms can creep so gradually into a woman's life that the changes are attributed to aging or stress.

▷ Symptoms are not consistent, even in the same person.

▷ When diseases of autoimmune origin arise, because they are at first specific to a particular organ, the patient is generally first referred to the (seemingly) appropriate medical specialist. For example, a patient with glandular problems might be sent by her internist to an endocrinologist. A hematologist may be called to evaluate diseases of the blood, and someone with neurological problems will be dispatched with haste to a neurologist. The rheumatologist (who specializes in autoimmune diseases) is often the last specialist anyone thinks of at the start of autoimmune-related symptoms.

Physicians unfamiliar with autoimmune diseases quite often will send patients away undiagnosed (or refer them to a psychiatrist, or put them on tranquilizers) because their symptoms—fatigue and pain, for example—are immeasurable and nonspecific. This is particularly a problem with diseases such as *fibromyalgia* and *chronic fatigue syndrome* (CFS), which, while not considered an autoimmune disease, may in fact herald an autoimmune disease.

One of the reasons that fibromyalgia and CFS, among other diseases, are not currently considered autoimmune diseases is that no autoantibody in these conditions has been located and no chemical change or altered cell population has been identified. No matter; I strongly believe they belong to our field—first, because they are so commonly associated with the other autoimmune diseases, and second, because I am convinced that they are real and not some psychological aberration. I have no doubt that these diseases will someday provide very important clues to many other diseases of the immune system. I also am convinced that some of them could turn out to be autoimmune diseases, if we find the right antigens for the antibody.

For me, diagnosing an autoimmune disease, and in fact any disease, represents the most rewarding side of medicine. It requires a substantial amount of judgment, a heaping portion of scientific knowledge, and the creativity of an artist. The care given to the pronouncement "You have X" cannot be overestimated, because with that simple sentence, both the length and quality of a patient's life can be altered forever, even if you are wrong. A physician is as human as the patient sitting in front of him or her, and the diagnosis of a disease can have grave effects. Upon this decision lies the course of the patient's therapy and the eventual outcome of her life. To practice medicine is a sublime privilege, and providing a correct diagnosis is an obligation no physician should ever take lightly.

I approach a diagnosis as a detective who is collecting clues. It gets easier to find the clues if you do it often enough. And it can be fun. On my way to work on the New York subway, for example, I will stand in the car and diagnose four or five illnesses just by observing the people around me. For example, I look at the color and texture of their skin, which can portend good health or not, but I also look at whether or not men have traces of a beard. If they do not, perhaps they have *Klinefelter syndrome*, a common chromosomal anomaly in which a man has an extra X chromosome. This results in too little estrogen and androgen, and a minimal amount of facial hair, so that Klinefelter patients rarely, if ever, shave. I notice whether women or men have sparse hair, full hair, or no hair and can often diagnose *alopecia*, which is far different from male-pattern baldness. I look at a person's eyes to see if they are bloodshot, which tells me that the eyes may be very dry, that there is irritation, and they may have *uveitis*—an autoimmune eye disease—or a viral infection, particularly if one eye is bloodshot and the other one is not. Even a passenger's fingers, as they hold the center pole, can reveal so much. If their fingers or joints are swollen, and depending on which joints are swollen, I can tell if they have osteoarthritis or rheumatoid arthritis (in rheumatoid arthritis, the joints closest to the palm get inflamed, and in osteoarthritis, it is the joints nearest the fingernails that are affected). If the last digits on the fingers are deformed and the person has a scaly rash, I know it is arthritis caused by psoriasis. If the skin on the fingers is taut and shiny, a diagnosis of scleroderma would most likely be accurate. I also observe the way people hold on to the overhead bar. If they extend their arms, it tells me they have muscle strength. The majority of people with polymyositis or dermatomyositis (two muscle-related autoimmune diseases) cannot lift their arms above their shoulders. And I smell them. I can smell alcohol on someone's breath a mile away, and I can detect *ketoacids,* which produces a sweetish smell. This can be a sure sign of diabetes. Sir Arthur Conan Doyle, who was a physician as well as the creator of Sherlock Holmes, always said that a good diagnostician must use every one of his or her senses. In his books, he always employed smell, taste, touch, vision, and sound or lack of sound—recall the dog that did not bark—to help Sherlock Holmes identify the culprit.

Playing subway detective aside, clearly there is no substitute for sitting with a patient and taking her history. Actually, my diagnosis begins when a patient walks into my office. I note if she walks in with confidence, how strong her grip is when she shakes my hand. Is she alone or with a relative? Is there hope or despair in her eyes? I try to decide if she wants all the facts or just a minimum, if she understands what I am saying or not. You have to ask everything. Are you a good artist? Are you prematurely gray? Do you have any birthmarks? Are you left- or right-handed? Everything has relevance.

Handedness and artistic capabilities are important to the way the brain develops and subsequently the way the immune system develops, because the two are so closely related. A higher incidence of left handedness in people with autoimmune disease has been well documented. These people are good artists, are extremely good with numbers, and generally have good hand-eye coordination. For example, I look at a little girl who is a pitcher on a Little League team and she is almost always left handed or ambidextrous. Not so long ago, I attended a game where a little girl was pitching against my son, who was batting. She pitched lefty and could catch splendidly with either hand. I happened to be sitting next to her mother and said, "Boy, your daughter is really talented. Has she been this way all her life?"

The mother said, "I'm not sure. I have lupus and getting out has been really difficult for me, so I really haven't seen her play very much."

The offspring, particularly males, who are born to women with autoimmune disease, tend to have certain characteristics. Dyslexia is one. In the early 1980s, I conducted a study, the results of which were published in 1984 in the *Journal of Psychoneuroimmunology*. The study showed that if more than one woman in an immediate family has a disease such as lupus, 55 percent of her male offspring will be dyslexic. This does not mean the child will get autoimmune disease; rather it means that he or she will be more prone to some of these associated characteristics. In keeping with this expectation, when discussing a patient's history with her, I might ask:

"Do you have children?"
"Yes."
"Do you have boys?"
"Two."
"How many are left-handed?"
"One of them."

Then I ask: Is he prematurely gray? Is he dyslexic? Is he good with numbers? And the patient is absolutely amazed. "Gee, Dr. Lahita. How did you know?" Then I have to explain that the crystal ball on my desk is absolutely powerless. These are just scientific facts.

Once I have completed taking an extensive history from the patient, I perform a physical examination. The physical exam confirms (or denies) the conclusions I have begun to draw and puts me one step closer to making a diagnosis. I hope the laboratory tests that follow will corroborate my suspicions scientifically, but as I have said, these are not always the last word. Taken as a whole, diagnosing requires a little bit of poetry, a lot of observation, and a penchant for leaving no stone unturned. When you get it right, there is no feeling like it in the world.

Women and Autoimmune Disease

Autoimmune diseases are a special threat to women. They are among the ten leading causes of death among women in all age groups up to sixty-five. Statistically, women represent 75 percent of the cases nationwide. The list below shows the prevalence of female-to-male ratio of specific autoimmune diseases in the United States.

FEMALE TO MALE RATIOS IN AUTOIMMUNE DISEASES

Hashimoto's thyroiditis	50:1
Lupus	9:1
Sjögren's syndrome	9:1
Antiphospholipid syndrome	9:1
Primary biliary cirrhosis	9:1
Chronic active hepatitis	8:1
Graves' disease	7:1
Rheumatoid arthritis	4:1
Scleroderma	3:1
Myasthenia gravis	2:1
Multiple sclerosis	2:1
Idiopathic thrombocytopenic purpura	2:1

Women are diagnosed with autoimmune disease most frequently during the childbearing years, which leads us to believe that hormones may have a direct connection to autoimmunity. Certainly, hormones affect the severity of disease, but the actual reason for the gender preference in most of these diseases is not scientifically known. In chapter 1 I mentioned my theory about the finely tuned nature of women's immune systems. The theory takes on added weight because most autoimmune illnesses strike women before menopause, while a few—generally thyroid related—occur more frequently after menopause. Mysteriously, some diseases suddenly improve during pregnancy, with flare-ups occurring after delivery, while others get worse during pregnancy. Some conditions are defined in part by pregnancy, such as antiphospholipid syndrome, which is so directly related to pregnancy that one of its three defining symptoms is multiple miscarriage.

One of the more recent theories put forth on why so many more women than men have autoimmune disease involves the *chimeric cell*, which was first identified in humans with autoimmune disease by my colleague Dr. Lee Hansen in Seattle. I recently was a visiting professor at the Mayo Clinic as a guest of the Clinical Fellows in Rheumatology. There, Dr. Anne Reed, a pediatrician who specializes in autoimmune muscle diseases (myositis) of children, reminded me of the importance of this cell.

The chimera, much like the two-headed creature of mythology, is a cell that contains both self and foreign genes. A chimeric cell always begins its life in the body of one human being before being transferred to another. The most common source of this "nonself" cell is the mother's blood, which is transferred to the fetus before birth, when the circulations of mother and baby were intimately tied together. The chimeric cell can also be transferred from the fetus to the mother during the process of birth, or it may have entered the body as the result of a blood transfusion.

Remarkably, such cells have been found in people of late middle age, who presumably have had them floating benignly in their circulation for many years, read by the immune system as "self." Then, for some unknown reason, suddenly the immune system sees these cells as foreign and goes on the attack. The result is an immune response called *graft versus host disease* (GVH) that can cause a number of autoimmune diseases. Many cases of scleroderma, myositis, and probably other conditions follow this pattern of chimeric-induced GVH.

Factors that May Provoke Autoimmune Disease

▷ *Ethnicity and Geographic Location*

In addition to gender preference, it is not uncommon to find certain autoimmune diseases that favor certain ethnic groups. For example, lupus is more common in African-American and Hispanic women than in Caucasian women. Rheumatoid arthritis and scleroderma affect a higher percentage of the Native American population than the general U.S. population. More white women get antiphospholipid syndrome than do women from any other ethnic group. A recent statistic showed that more black than white women die of lupus-related kidney disease. Why? Nobody really knows, but one hypothesis is that it is because more black women live in poverty, and thus lack health insurance. Consequently, these women use clinics and the emergency room as their primary source of medical care, which means they do not have access to early diagnosis by a specialist and aggressive, early treatment, when warranted. It is also possible that a lack of health education, an unbalanced diet, and the general living conditions of the poorer people in this country render them more vulnerable. Is there a genetic component? Perhaps, but most autoimmune diseases have genetic associations with chromosome 6, which has nothing to do with a person's ethnicity.

People from different geographical areas have different kinds of responses, too. For example, a woman from a developing part of Africa is exposed daily to life-threatening bacterial infections and various parasites. If she moves to a more developed area, where she is treated on occasion with antibiotics, she might then be deprived of her natural immunity, and her immune system would have the potential to overreact. This is the theory of *antigen exposure*. In other words, black people from Africa may get lupus less often than black people who move to America, because antigen exposure in Africa protects them from such autoimmune problems. When they move, their exposure to a high-tech, noninfectious society might actually be detrimental to their immune systems. The theory stating that black women who come to America from Africa contract lupus more often than those who stay in Africa has been cited often but not adequately explained. I mention it here only because I have heard it so many times. I am not sure that it is true, or, perhaps, in Africa they are just not diagnosing lupus as often as they might.

▷ **Genetic Connections**

There is no question that genetics play a role in the development of autoimmune disease. Women, and men for that matter, definitely can inherit genes that contribute to the susceptibility for developing an autoimmune disease. Certain diseases, psoriasis, for example, cluster in members of the same family, which suggests that a specific gene or set of genes predisposes members of that family to the skin disorder. Then, too, particular members of a family can develop completely different autoimmune diseases, which means they have a propensity toward autoimmune disease in general, but not to a specific disease. This is most apparent in large families in which the same genes exist on chromosome 6 (the location of the immune response genes), but not all of the children get autoimmune diseases. If several children do get autoimmune diseases, they may not all get the same disease. In the case of identical twins in which the two siblings share identical genes, the likelihood of both twins getting the same disease ranges from 2 percent to 25 percent. This tells us that even in identical twins, there are predispositions, but there is no *Mendelian* model (if you have the gene, you get the disease) for these illnesses.

▷ *Environmental Factors*

Environmental factors and lifestyle habits clearly can provoke the immune system. As mentioned in the last chapter, chronic alcoholism results in a state of weakened immunity. Alcoholics who succumb to infections usually do so because the chronic poisoning of the body by the drug alcohol weakens their immune systems. Certain medical treatments also can be at fault. Chemotherapy, a knight in shining armor when it comes to treating cancer, can turn into a miscreant at other times. Long before we knew about AIDS, I was a resident at the Sloan Kettering Cancer Center in New York and saw the kinds of infections that we now see in AIDS patients happening in patients on heavy chemotherapy for cancer, such as *Pneumocystis carinii*, which lives in the normal lung as a harmless resident. The terrible infections we see in AIDS patients—"bread mold" pneumonia, *Nocardiosis*, another type of mold; variants of TB; and pneumocystis carinii—give an idea of how important the immune system is in protecting us from harmless common organisms in our environment.

▷ *Stress*

Stress can provoke new autoimmune disease and often worsens existing autoimmune disease in ways we do not fully understand. Many scientific studies have shown that immune cells drop in numbers when an animal or a person is subjected to severe stress. I have personally known patients who suffer severe setbacks in their diseases when they are exposed to stresses such as a death in the family or a divorce. The area of stress-induced disease is now a field of study called *psychoneuroimmunology*.

Treating Autoimmune Diseases

Because most autoimmune diseases are chronic, most patients must be monitored and treated for life. With good treatment, however, many people can and do live normal lives. Since at present there is no cure for these diseases, for now the standard as well as the most innovative treatment is aimed at lessening the severity of symptoms.

Prescribing drugs for patients with autoimmune disease is one of those components in medical practice, like diagnosis, in which the physician's prowess improves with experience. Experience matters a great deal in treating autoimmune diseases because there are so many diseases and because each disease has so many integral components. Most drugs are aimed at helping patients manage the consequences of inflammation caused by the autoimmune disease. People with type 1 diabetes can suffer damage to their eyes, kidneys, and blood vessels if their blood sugar levels rise too far from an acceptable range so medications must include insulin to keep blood sugar levels in control. In diseases such as lupus or rheumatoid arthritis, corticosteroids are often prescribed to slow down or even suppress the immune system response in an attempt to curtail often-debilitating symptoms. Chemotherapy drugs such as cyclophosphamide or nitrogen mustard are used to treat autoimmune diseases as well. They are generally employed in far lower concentration than for cancer, however, because the objective is not to obliterate a tumor but rather to fine-tune the immune response. These and other more specific treatments are discussed in more depth in each chapter and in the chapter on drugs at the end of the book.

While suppressing the immune system chemically has its benefits, it also has its drawbacks. A compromised (or suppressed) immune system, while decreasing symptoms, may open the door to infection in the body and other potentially serious side effects. This is why it is so important to work with a highly experienced physician. In some people, immunosuppressive medications may result in disease remission, but even so, these same patients generally remain on the medication because to discontinue it might bring on symptoms again.

Research tells us that in women, estrogens stimulate the immune system, and that male hormones, androgens, have the reverse effect. So it would follow that in autoimmune disease, in which the immune system is running rampant, the way to slow disease progression is to give a patient male hormones. While many physicians do precisely this, I personally am skeptical because, in truth, the effects are so minor that I am not sure it makes much difference. Still, I do offer testosterone on rare occasions. because in some cases there appears to be some benefit, and anything that helps—for example, by increasing memory or providing more energy—is worth a try. These hormones make no change in the overall severity of the illness, however, at least none that I have ever seen.

The major reason I do not believe male hormones are very effective in treating women is that I am convinced the immune system, like the brain, is fixed or imprinted before birth, and I doubt that any kind of hormonal manipulation can change what is already programmed. This concept, which is called imprinting or *sexing*, means that hormones present before birth produce irreversible marks on the cells. This flies in the face of convention; many researchers believe to the contrary. But if I believed that male hormones suppressed the immune system and could reverse autoimmune disease, I would give testosterone to all my sick patients, which I do not do.

Because every patient is different, every disease is different, and every symptom is subjective, there is no way to predict a course of events based on either how the disease starts or the depth of the symptoms. A good physician recognizes the importance of closely monitoring his or her patients. Patients, for their part, must keep to a schedule of frequent visits to the physician so that he or she can manage complex treatment regimens and watch for side effects from the medications. With autoimmune disease, as indeed with any disease, it is very important to have a good rapport with your physician; you are going to be associates for a very long time.

AIDS versus Autoimmunity: A Short Lesson

AIDS is a disease of the immune system, but it is not an autoimmune disease. I am including this discussion because so many people confuse the two diseases, and it is important to understand the difference. In patients with autoimmune disease, the immune system is working overtime; immune cells are multiplying rampantly in an effort to destroy what is perceived to be a foreign invader. In patients with AIDS, which stands for *acquired immune deficiency syndrome*, the immune system itself is the target of a virus—the human immunodeficiency virus (HIV)—and after the attack, the immune system is severely compromised, leaving the patient open to severe infection and possibly cancer. One of the curious aspects of AIDS is that early on in the infection, the T helper cells are stimulated and many autoantibodies are made. In fact, during the first months of HIV, many patients may be confused as those with autoimmunity. Once the CD4 cells—T cells that usually boost immune function—begin to die after infection, the autoantibodies disappear.

I have a great interest in AIDS because I was present in the early eighties when the disease was being described for the first time as Gay-Related Immunodeficiency Disease, or GRID. I was at the Rockefeller University, mouth pipetting (suctioning blood partially up into a tiny glass tube), and drawing blood without gloves from patients with GRID so that we could study this immunodeficiency in the lab. At the time, no one had any idea that this was a viral illness. It was only known that the disease caused a depletion of immune strength. What I, and indeed all of us in the labs, did was tantamount to what Osler and Ehrlich did in their day, when they performed autopsies on bodies without wearing rubber gloves, all in the name of science. But what did we, or they, know?

The Future of Autoimmune Disease Treatment

First, the bad news: To date, there is no cure for autoimmune diseases. Now, the good news: *So far*. We are working on it. Rest assured that for every autoimmune disease, there is a laboratory—perhaps hundreds of laboratories—with a group of scientists hunched over computers, calibrating test tubes, looking through microscopes at cells, and analyzing genes and molecules in an attempt to define their roles. Some of these scientists are seeking treatments that produce remissions with fewer side effects. Others are developing therapies that target various steps in the immune response. Still others are examining new approaches, such as the use of therapeutic antibodies against specific T-cell molecules. The hope here is that the therapeutic antibodies might produce fewer long-term side effects than the chemotherapies that now are routinely used. Currently, significant time and resources are spent studying the immune system itself and pathways of inflammation. Ultimately, of course, the goal is to prevent autoimmune diseases altogether.

At the beginning of this chapter, I showed how our concepts of autoimmunity reached adolescence during the 1970s and 1980s. Now, with decades of research behind us, these concepts are still maturing. The deluge of scientific knowledge that comes our way daily and the newer insights into diseases that previously were not considered autoimmune have convinced me that finding a cure is not all that different from the early concept of landing on the moon. It is only a matter of time, because it is out there. I know it is. I can almost see it.

PART TWO

The Autoimmune Diseases

CHAPTER THREE

THE ANTIPHOSPHOLIPID SYNDROME

⌒

Sticky Blood

ONE DAY SEVERAL years ago, Barbara and a few of her classmates were crossing the Columbia University campus when, without warning, she found herself sitting on the grass. "Literally," she later told me. "My leg just buckled. One moment I was up and the next one I was down." Her friends were just as surprised as she was. Together, they looked for something Barbara might have tripped over or stepped into, but found nothing. A bit bewildered, she attributed the incident to clumsiness and continued on to lunch with the group. Barbara didn't know it at the time, but as she and her friends headed along the path toward the cafeteria, deep inside her body her antibodies had just dealt the first blow in what soon would become a very devastating illness.

Several weeks later, the incident completely forgotten, Barbara awoke from a nap to find her left leg twitching uncontrollably in spasmodic jerks. This lasted several seconds; then, as she started to get up, she felt a sharp pain in her head. The headache would turn out to be the first of many migraines to come. Barbara's roommate handed her three aspirin and convinced her that she was fortunate to have gone so long without ever having had that type of debilitating headache. " 'Count your lucky stars,' " is the way she put it," Barbara later explained. "And so I guess I did."

With the headache behind her and the twitching leg incident forgotten, Barbara settled in to study for final exams. When they were over, however, she began to notice something new: Her clothes felt tight, particularly two skirts she had only recently purchased. A dreaded trip to the scale confirmed her suspicion of weight gain. Less than thrilled, she rationalized it away, telling herself that it was because she had stopped jogging. There was no time, with finals and all. Besides, who can run with a leg you can no longer count on? (Her leg had acted up a few more times.) "In retrospect," she told me at our first meeting, "if they gave out medals in denial, I would have belonged right up there at the front of the line."

Barbara's varying symptoms continued, sporadically at times, sometimes subtly, sometimes not so subtly. She had several more migraines, an episode of shortness of breath, and more fleeting leg tremors. Then one morning, about six weeks after the first signs had appeared, Barbara began to cough. At first the cough was dry, but within hours, blood-tinged specks appeared on the tissue, and very soon after, she was coughing up tiny clots. "You know, Dr. Lahita," she told me later, "you can only deny so much. I guess I was waiting for someone to throw a sandbag at me to wake me up. With those little clots on the tissue, I had finally met my Waterloo."

Barbara made an appointment to see her general physician at noon the next day, but that morning, she woke up with her leg so swollen she found it almost impossible to walk. With the help of a friend, she made it to the college infirmary where the nurse very wisely sent her directly to the hospital emergency room.

When I first saw Barbara that afternoon in the ER, she had already been there for several hours. She was in a private examining room, one of three in the twenty-bed unit. I found a pale young woman with dark circles around her frightened eyes, lying on a narrow bed, arms clasped across her chest. My first thought was that she looked like a teenage girl in need of her mother. The nurses had already exchanged her clothes for a hospital gown—her jeans and sweatshirt were on a chair near the door—and although we had not yet met, she seemed relieved when I approached the examining table.

"Are you the specialist?" she asked.

"I am, and I think we're both very lucky that Dr. Knoll knew to call me," I said, indicating the physician in blue scrubs across from me. Dr. Knoll was the chief resident in emergency medicine who, quite serendipitously, had attended one of my lectures the week before. In a teaching hospital, every attending physician is required to deliver a minimum number of talks to the house staff, and on that day my lecture had been on autoimmune diseases and their mysterious manifestations. Clearly, Dr. Knoll was paying close attention, because when he examined Barbara and heard her symptoms, he had, as he put it, "a feeling of déjà vu." He was absolutely right. Barbara did indeed turn out to have an autoimmune disease, though not vasculitis, which was the one I had used as the illustrative example in my lecture. Still, were I giving out grades, I would give him an A for the day. He just might have saved this woman's life.

Dr. Knoll told me that when he first saw Barbara and examined her swollen leg, his initial thought was that she might have a *phlebitis* (inflammation of the blood vessel as the result of a lodged blood clot), and so he quickly started her on heparin, an anticoagulant that would immediately thin her blood and prevent further clots.

There are two classifications of blood clots: A stationary clot, which is usually lodged against the inner wall of a blood vessel, is called a *thrombus*. A clot that breaks away and travels down the bloodstream is called an *embolus*. If Barbara indeed had a clot, she needed urgent treatment in case the clot broke away from the side of the vessel and traveled to her lung, blocking the circulation to the lung and subsequently the flow of blood to the heart—a condition known as pulmonary embolus. Blood clots to the heart, the brain, or the lung can be deadly. In 50 percent of reported cases of coronary artery disease, where a clot lodges in a narrowed coronary artery, cutting off the blood supply to the heart, the very first symptom is sudden death. The same might be said for a pulmonary embolus, which is what took the life of the young reporter David Bloom during the 2003 Iraqi war. One split second and you're down.

I immediately examined Barbara's leg and found it to be red, swollen, and warm to the touch, which told me that the blood flow was not severely hindered and that the chances were not likely that a clot was occurring in one of the arteries or veins that supplied the entire lower leg. Had that been the case, her leg would have been cold and blue. Swollen, red, and edematous (fluid-filled) indicate a venous clot—or a phlebitis. From the subtle but striated pattern of vessels that were slightly raised, I suspected that she did not have a deep venous thrombosis, but rather a variety of smaller clots in the deep veins. That was actually good news; it also bought us some time. As the heparin dripped into her wrist, and with all her vital signs now stable, I pulled up a chair and listened as she described the history of her symptoms. When the words "weight gain, migraine, leg tremors, shortness of breath, coughing up blood, overall fatigue," were woven through her story, although there was a long way to go to prove it, I had a feeling we were looking at *antiphospholipid syndrome* (APLS), a disorder that, at its very best, is highly treatable and at its worst can be catastrophic.

What Is Antiphospholipid Syndrome?

APLS is a disorder that affects the clotting properties of the blood. It can occur in the primary form, meaning without other autoimmune disorders, or in the secondary form, when it happens in patients with other diseases, most notably lupus.

Phospholipids are molecules that are present on the surface of most of the cells in the body. They are responsible for helping blood clot when it needs to. They also make up a good part of the surface of the platelet, which is necessary for clot formation. Platelets are not cells, but rather fragments that float in the blood and clump together to help form clots any time the blood needs to clot, such as after something as minor as a paper cut, or as major as an invasive operation or a serious injury. APLS results when the immune system sees phospholipids as foreign and produces antibodies against them.

Essentially, when antibodies form against phospholipids, they are forming against two different entities: clotting factors and platelets. When the clotting factor is the target, that factor is altered so that the blood clots in ways that it is not intended to. After being assaulted by antibodies, clots begin to appear in unnatural places, places where they can cause problems, such as along the walls of veins and arteries where their presence disturbs the flow of blood.

When antiphospholipid antibodies attack platelets, which normally help form clots, they change the surface of the platelets. Platelets coated with antibody tend to become tacky and ultimately begin to stick to each other in clumps, rendering them completely useless. This is why APLS has been given the name "sticky blood syndrome"—for sticky cells, sticky clots, and clumping platelets.

Possible Causes of Antiphospholipid Syndrome

Why was Barbara fine one minute and so very ill the next? What caused her disease? No one knows for sure. It is thought that APLS is most likely caused by an infection. Some researchers have shown that parts of organisms, such as the walls of a bacterial cell or the coatings of viruses, are especially reactive with the antiphospholipid antibodies. It would not surprise me to find that some rogue virus confused the immune system and provoked it to attack the phospholipids. In addition, APLS may run in families, although it is not necessarily inherited. I wish there were more to explain, but not much more is known about the etiology of this disease, which we have been aware of for only twenty years—not a very long time in the overall framework of medicine. To date there are still many more questions than answers.

The Three Components of Antiphospholipid Syndrome

APLS is often called Hughes syndrome, after my English colleague, Graham Hughes, who contributed to our understanding of one of the great medical puzzles of this specialty. In 1983 Dr. Hughes and his wonderful team of Drs. Harris, Gharavi, Asherson, and Khamashta, from St. Thomas Hospital in London, described a complex clinical syndrome characterized by *thrombosis* (blood clots), *thrombocytope-nia* (low platelets often leading to internal bleeding), and *recurrent miscarriage*.

Although many patients with those syndromes fell under the general heading of lupus, or lupus-like disease, the people Dr. Hughes and his colleagues described had phospholipid antibodies but did not meet the criteria for having lupus. Even though lupus is the disorder with which APLS is most closely associated in terms of symptoms, Hughes found the group to be sufficiently different from those with typical systemic lupus to warrant separate categorization. (I should mention that patients with APLS often do develop lupus.) Today we still use Dr. Hughes's triple categorization to describe APLS. Let us take a look at each of these components separately.

▷ Thrombosis

A thrombosis is a blood clot that can arise in any of the small, medium, or large veins or arteries that comprise the circulatory system. In APLS, it is the result of antibody reacting against clotting factor. Depending on where the thrombosis lodges, the aftermath can be of minor consequence, quite serious, or even fatal. Here are some of the locations where a thrombus can settle and the consequences that ensue:

- ▷ Heart—myocardial infarction, coronary artery disease, valvular disease.
- ▷ Kidney or renal artery—malignant hypertension, vasculitis.
- ▷ Glands—Addison's disease.
- ▷ Reproductive system—recurrent miscarriage.
- ▷ Bloodstream—autoimmune hemolytic anemia.
- ▷ Lungs—adult respiratory distress syndrome, pulmonary hypertension, pulmonary embolus.
- ▷ Eyes—blurry vision, transient field loss, changes in the retina and optic nerve.
- ▷ Brain—transient ischemic attack (small stroke), venous thrombosis, epilepsy, Guillain-Barré syndrome, migraine headache, and chorea (small, jerky movements of the limbs).

▷ Ovarian and uterine veins—infertility, loss of ovary, blockage of circulation to the uterus.

▷ Legs and arm veins—deep vein thrombosis or, if superficial, superficial thrombosis or phlebitis.

▷ *Thrombocytopenia*

When associated with APLS, thrombocytopenia results when antibodies react with the surface of the platelets. This condition by itself yields symptoms that are the *opposite* of clotting. Thrombocytopenia generates bleeding and often hemorrhaging. Remember, it takes platelets to make clots. A normal platelet count is 150,000 to 300,000. In someone with thrombocytopenia, the count can drop precipitously to about 20,000. As the level of working platelets drops, the patient begins to develop bruising all over. I admit to getting nervous when a patient's platelet count goes below 15,000, because if the platelets get any lower, the patient can spontaneously bleed into the head and end up with a stroke.

Low platelet counts also occur in the autoimmune disease *idiopathic thrombocytopenic purpura* (ITP), which is what strikes poor Bea in chapter 4. The circumstances of both antiphospholipid thrombocytopenia and ITP are the same—low or nonexistent platelets—but ITP is characterized *only* by low platelets. With APLS, you can have low platelets *and* the propensity to clot at the same time.

You may be wondering, How can one have both low platelets *and* the propensity to clot? A good question. We have just seen that the antibody against phospholipid does two things: It reacts with clotting factors, leading to changes on the cell surface that cause it to stick together and form clots, and at the same time, it might react toward the platelets and wipe them out, with a good possibility of excessive bleeding. Therefore, an unfortunate individual who has both an antibodies to a clotting factor *and* the propensity to clot can both hemorrhage and clot at the same time.

When I think of bleeding and clotting at the same time in a patient with APLS, I cannot help but remember what happened with a patient of mine with APLS who did just that, although his bleeding occurred as a result of his taking an anticoagulant, rather than by his disease. This thirty-two-year-old man had come to see me six weeks before Thanksgiving with deep vein thrombosis resulting from APLS. He had antibodies to many clotting factors and was clotting in some parts of his body, so I placed him on an anticoagulant to keep more clots from forming. Basically, I thinned his blood. I later heard from his wife that at Thanksgiving dinner, he choked on some food, and a cousin at the table rushed over and performed the Heimlich maneuver. In the process, he ruptured my patient's liver and he hemorrhaged to death, right there at the Thanksgiving table, because he had no way of clotting his blood. This is not exactly a beautiful image, but the next time someone asks you whether it is possible to have thin blood and clots simultaneously, I have a feeling you will remember the answer.

▷ Multiple Miscarriages

This is the third and, for young women, perhaps most distressing condition that stems from APLS. It is not clear how or why, but we know for sure that APLS can have devastating effects on pregnant women. Women with this disease have difficulty in both conceiving their babies and carrying them to term, which is why it is becoming a major concern among both reproductive endocrinologists and obstetricians.

A common early theory linking APLS to miscarriage was that microscopic blood clots arose and lodged in the blood vessels of the placenta, narrowing or blocking the vessels, thereby depriving the fetus of oxygen and nutrients, and ultimately hastening a miscarriage. But we now know from animal experiments that the antibody itself can actually be poisonous to the placenta—to the degree that the woman might reject the placenta. It may actually be a little of both, but I believe the toxic antibody effect is likely to be the most important mechanism.

APLS can have other serious effects, too. For example, the risk in mothers may include stroke, clots, hypertension, stillbirths, recurrent miscarriage, poor fetal growth, and preterm delivery. Pregnancy loss can occur at any time during the gestational period, but occurrence in the second or third trimester is most characteristic. According to a statistic from the Cincinnati Children's Hospital, as many as 33 percent of women with APLS deliver before thirty-two weeks' gestation.

I have seen APLS sufferers who have had as many as fourteen consecutive miscarriages. That they wait so long to get a proper diagnosis is clearly understandable, however, because not all obstetricians know to look for it. But that they continue to try to produce a child, that they show such resiliency of spirit in such difficult circumstances, is one of the main characteristics in women that keep me in awe.

Pregnant women with APLS have the best chance of carrying to term if they keep in very close contact with their obstetricians so that the pregnancy can be closely monitored and ultrasounds can be administered to watch the fetus's growth. Treatment, which includes low-dose baby aspirin administered from the beginning of the pregnancy until just before delivery, has proven to be very successful in helping a woman carry her baby to term. In women who have suffered earlier miscarriages, heparin (a blood thinner) or even prednisone (an immunosuppresive) combined with baby aspirin may be used.

Although there are a few reports of successful pregnancies without treatment, the majority of researchers have reported a 70 to 75 percent success rate with treatment. Close observation and delivering the baby at the first signs of fetal distress has been the most successful formula for having a healthy baby when the mother has APLS.

Diagnosing Antiphospholipid Syndrome

When I suspect a patient has APLS, I first do a complex history and physical and then follow with the appropriate tests to prove or disprove my suspicions. Each aspect of the diagnosis is of the utmost importance, but in most cases I find the history is the most invaluable. There is so much to be learned. Here is the process I used to reach my conclusion with Barbara:

▷ *History*

As Barbara reported the events leading up to her arrival at the hospital, I knew that the inflamed venous patterns on her legs and the coughing up of blood were due to the migration of thousands of small clots to her lower left leg and to her lungs. This was my first clue that she had a condition in which her blood was much too thick.

The issue of slow and steady weight gain, particularly after she told me her eating habits had not changed, indicated that she might have glandular involvement. The most common gland involved in this type of behavior is the thyroid gland. I surmised that Barbara's weight gain was symptomatic of underactive or *hypothyroid* function, in all likelihood an effect of or even one of the reasons for this autoimmune disease. Autoimmune thyroid disease often accompanies other immune-related conditions or can exist on its own, as you will see in chapter 3.

Migraines, such as those Barbara experienced, are often found in young women with APLS and are of unknown cause. In fact, a migraine is often the first symptom of APLS. The tremors and involuntary movements of her leg, called *chorea,* were probably indicative of antibody activity against the cells of the brain. This is one of the enigmas of this syndrome—the direct toxic effects of the antibodies on the brain itself. Other neurological manifestations can include stroke, epilepsy, and myelopathy (muscle inflammation).

▷ *Physical Examination*

On examining Barbara, the first thing I looked for was APLS-related *livedo reticularis,* which is a marbleization of the skin, usually on the arms and thighs and over the knees. Because this symptom is more prominent in cold weather, I always crank up the air conditioners in my examining room to try to produce it, but I didn't need to do this in the ER. It was evident. Then, I felt her lower calf for *cords,* which are a series of clots within the vein that produce a ropelike feeling when you rub your finger over it. The presence of even a single cord generally indicates deep vein thrombosis.

Next, I pulled out my stethoscope and listened to her heart sounds. I heard a very loud heart murmur over the left side of her chest, which I knew indicated a problem with the mitral valve. The mitral valve consists of two gentle flaps, attached by tiny muscles that open and close. It is the first portal of entry for oxygen-filled blood from the lungs. When the flaps do not open properly, blood cannot easily flow through from one chamber to the next and so it begins to back up in the lungs. APLS can be associated with "vegetation" that grows on the heart valves. Fortunately, it is not common in a patient with this condition. These vegetations are not really alive or infectious; they are simply clumps of clotting material that hang off the valve.

I was also concerned about her leg movements and wanted to know whether this was truly an involuntary movement or some form of seizure. As she did not have a tremor when I was examining her, I decided to order an MRI of her head. This revealed a number of demyelinated (denuded) areas in her brain, but thankfully no strokes. Demyelination, or loss of insulation around the nerves of the brain, can be observed with any number of autoimmune diseases, but it is the major cause of symptoms associated with multiple sclerosis (MS). In fact, it is often difficult to differentiate other causes of demyelination from MS. This is where the art of medicine becomes so important. When demyelination attends APLS, that tells me that the antibody attacking the phospholipids is also attacking the common proteins of the myelin sheath and wreaking havoc in the brain.

Barbara did not have deep vein thrombosis (DVT), which is common in APLS, but when a patient does, I generally will confirm these findings with a Doppler study of the lower extremities. A Doppler is an ultrasound test that is based on the same technology that was used to seek out submarines in World War II. We bounce sound waves off of the patient's blood vessels and listen for a dull sound, which indicates that there is a clot in the blood vessel, blocking the flow of blood. Finally, just to be certain I am correct, I will do a Homan's test. This consists of grabbing the patient's toes and pushing back forcefully on the foot. The process stretches the Achilles tendon and cramps the calf. If the patient cries out in pain, I know I have a positive Homan's sign, which is helpful in confirmation of a deep vein thrombosis, if not exactly pleasing to the patient.

▷ *Laboratory Tests*

After assessing Barbara's clinical signs and finding them positive, I next sought out the presence of antiphospholipid antibodies, particularly the more common ones: *anticardiolipin* and *lupus anticoagulant*. (Strangely, lupus anticoagulant has nothing to do with lupus in most cases, nor is it an anticoagulant. Actually, it is a *pro*coagulant, because it encourages clotting. This was one of those things that were named inappropriately, and the name, for whatever reason, was never changed.)

One of the interesting things about cardiolipin and other phospholipids is that they are antigens that can show up on the valve of the heart. They also find a home in the inner membranes of what is called *Treponema pallidum*, the syphilis organism—which is why so many people with APLS falsely test positive for syphilis. This is not always without consequence. Several years ago, I had a patient who was an Orthodox Jew from a Hasidic family in Brooklyn. A year before she came to see me, she and the man she was to marry (it was an arranged marriage) went to City Hall, with his parents in tow, to obtain the marriage license. The couple brought with them the results of their required blood tests. The results showed that the bride-to-be was positive for syphilis, and the license was not granted. "This is impossible!" she told the furious groom and his enraged father. "I'm a virgin!" She was retested several times and still the results came back positive. His father did not believe her and canceled the wedding. She ended up in my office a year later with APLS, the symptoms of which had just become apparent. When I explained the situation to her, she was very relieved on two accounts. First, of course, she was glad to be able to clear up the mystery behind her positive syphilis tests, and second, because she never went through with the arranged marriage. It turns out she never liked the guy anyway. Eventually she married someone else. The moral? There are some good things that can result from this disease.

Barbara tested positive for both anticardiolipin and lupus anticoagulant, and so the diagnosis was assuredly APLS. Now all that was left was to treat her disease and get her back to school as soon as possible. Fortunately for all of us, this is one of the easier autoimmune conditions to deal with.

Treating Antiphospholipid Syndrome

When I went in to see Barbara on the third day after her admission to the hospital, she seemed much improved. The look of concern she had worn the past two days was replaced by one of self-assurance. Her room was overflowing with stuffed animals and flowers and she was busily chatting with two friends, both of whom were perched on the windowsill. The swelling in her leg was on its way down, and she was clearly more comfortable and alert than she had been the past two days. She gave me a big welcoming smile. "What's the final verdict, doctor?" she asked. "Am I going to be good as new?"

I could safely assure her she would. For all the destruction it can perpetrate on the body, antiphospholipid syndrome is easily treated with anticoagulants to thin the blood and inhibit the clots. End of story. Well, maybe not the end of the story, but certainly close. Sometimes the patient requires immunosuppressive drugs to keep the T cells in line when they get out of control, but those drugs are generally prescribed only as needed. A continual controversy at many of the scientific meetings of autoimmune specialists—one that will come up again at the Lupus Congress in 2004—is whether patients should only be given anticoagulants or should also be immunosuppressed. Half the immunology world feels they should be simultaneously placed on immunosuppressive drugs; the other half are proponents of anticoagulants only. I personally do not add immunosuppressants unless there is vasculitis or an ulcer of the skin, or even uveitis of the eyeball, a condition in which the patient is losing sight.

I started Barbara on heparin while she was in the hospital and discharged her on Coumadin, which has a different mode of action than heparin and is taken orally. Now, several months later, she is thriving on a combination of the Coumadin and a daily baby aspirin. Taken together, these two drugs prevent the clumping of platelets, which keeps her headaches and her involuntary leg movements at bay. As I had suspected, her weight gain was indeed attributed to a condition called *thyroiditis*—inflammation of the thyroid gland caused by the autoantibody (see chapter 13). That gland was an additional target for the immune system and was actually in the process of being rejected when she first came into the hospital. As her thyroid continued to be underactive and sluggish, Barbara began taking a thyroid medication called Synthroid to replace what hormone was lost. Even her cough cleared up, which indicates that she has stopped showering her lungs with clots.

Barbara might have to have her blood thinned for the rest of her life or at least until we understand this illness a little better. She knows she can never smoke, nor can she take estrogen, both of which tend to promote blood clots, but she agrees that it is a small price to pay for the relief of symptoms.

What happened to Barbara was a reminder that we are all human beings and no matter how young we are, how great we feel, or how glorious the day, we all fall to the ground once in a while. We are part of the world of nature. We are, as Lewis Thomas calls us, a fragile species, "only tentatively set in place, error prone, at risk of fumbling . . ."

CHAPTER FOUR

IDIOPATHIC THROMBOCYTOPENIC PURPURA

Murder in the Village: The Case of the Homicidal Antibody

T THE RISK of sounding like some two-bit pulp fiction novelist, it really was a dark and stormy night. I had just sat down for dinner when my plectron went off. A plectron is a beeper that calls the local ambulance corps, police, and firefighters in the village where I live. I am a volunteer member of the rescue squad in my village, and because I am a physician, I serve as the Emergency Medical Service (EMS) medical director and the police and fire surgeon as well. I have done this for twelve years, but since my hours are so long at the hospital, I have arranged to be called only to the most serious situations—those involving people who are unconscious, in cardiac arrest, or victims of major motor-vehicle accidents or choking. On the night in question the call came over as an "unconscious and unresponsive" and gave the precise address. I put down my fork, jumped into my car, and arrived at that address within minutes. There it was that I came upon a most memorable scene of chaos and mayhem.

Pulling up in front of the house, I noted a series of cars that told me the EMTs (emergency medical technicians) were already on the premises. (Unlike paramedics, EMTs are trained volunteers whose day jobs may be of a completely different nature.) Three police officers crowded together on the small front porch, and one headed to my car to fill me on the details while I drew my bag from the trunk. Within minutes, an ambulance came to a halt across the street, and two paramedics dashed past me into the house. I followed them in great haste, and as I did so, I saw through the dim light of the hallway the body of an unconscious young woman, nude from the waist down, lying on the floor. Two EMTs were kneeling on either side of her. They told me they had been summoned by a neighbor and had found the woman sprawled on the bathroom floor. They had found it necessary to move her several feet into the hallway to have room enough to tend to her. I noticed that her pajama top was open and the med techs were doing CPR. As the ranking medical officer, I immediately took charge.

The paramedics assisted me as I gave the patient adrenalin to try to restore electrical activity to her heart. She was already hooked up to an EKG (electrocardiograph), and an IV was in place in her left wrist. As CPR continued, one of the paramedics knelt at the woman's head, angled it back, and slid a breathing tube into her trachea in order to infuse a high concentration of oxygen into her lungs to sustain the oxygen content in her blood. CPR continued all the while as we frantically tried to get back some life, but the woman did not respond. Her EKG was flat; her heart had stopped, and after twenty minutes of resuscitative efforts it became apparent we were getting nowhere. I decided to pronounce her dead, which I do by simply looking at my watch, noting the time, and saying, "It is such-and-such a time. This woman is deceased."

Before I make a pronouncement, I routinely do several things, all of which I attended to in this case: I check the patient's pupils, listen to the heart and chest, and do a cursory examination to be sure there are no holes in the body from bullets, knives, or other sources. In order to do so, I edged my way past the paramedic to where her head was in order to get a better look. I asked the officer nearby for a flashlight, because the hallway had so little light. He handed me a searchlight, which I directed toward her face. Pulling back an eyelid, I saw that her pupils were fixed and dilated, which, not surprisingly, indicated that the woman was dead. But what did surprise me were the *petechiae*. I noted a scattering of tiny small hemorrhages around her pupils, which suggested to me that she had suffered some sort of anoxia (absence of oxygen). I last saw petechiae in the eyes of a young girl who had earlier, and most tragically, been strangled. I should mention that as a student in medical school, I worked alongside the medical examiner, Dr. Milton Halperin, in New York, so I was most familiar with strangulations, murders, ligature hangings, and stabbings. I can safely say, from experience, that one does not see petechiae in a person's eyes unless they have been strangled, or at least I never had. I then pulled the light in tighter to examine her face, and the rest of her body. On close examination, I noted four blue marks across the front and sides of her neck, almost as if fingers had been placed there. Curious, I asked the paramedic to turn her over, and there we all beheld an area of hemorrhaging under the skin around her buttocks and blood around her anus. The paramedic, seeing it for the first time as I was, said, "Doc, are you thinking what I'm thinking? You think this lady was sodomized?" It certainly seemed like a good possibility.

Putting the neck marks together with the eye hemorrhages and the bloody anus, all signs pointed to foul play. I turned to the police officer next to me and said in my most Hercule Poirotian voice: "Seal off the house! This is a crime scene!" Then two of the police officers began roping off everything in yellow-crime-scene tape while the third officer called on his radio for reinforcements. The next thing I knew, even more police officers, detectives, the medical examiner (ME), one very nervous pathologist, and a teenage-looking reporter from the local newspaper, descended upon us. Remember, this is a very small village.

The homicide detectives moved the EMTs, the paramedics, and me into the side rooms to debrief us and to allow them to more easily inspect the crime area. They gave us booties to cover our shoes, and gloves so we wouldn't leave fingerprints anywhere, which made no sense to us, because we had already mucked up the whole place trying to resuscitate the poor woman. I went into the kitchen to find one detective talking to the neighbor who had made the emergency call. She told us the victim's name was Bea G. She said she had seen the victim's car in the driveway earlier, and saw lights on in the house, so she walked over to return a cake plate. After knocking on the door and getting no reply, she opened it and called in. It was then that she heard the moans from the bathroom and dialed 911.

As I was getting ready to leave, I passed by the hallway where the medical examiner was completing his examination of the body by taking swabs of the affected areas and putting them into small glass vials. He said that he, too, believed this was most definitely a homicide and would contact me as soon as he learned something. As I got into my car, I saw the techs from the medical examiner's office wheeling the woman through the rain toward their van. She was zippered up in a generic morgue bag—now just another ill-fated homicide victim.

Early the next morning, my telephone rang. It was the ME's assistant.

"Doc?"
"Yes?"
"We found the culprit."
"You found him already?"
"There was no *him*, Doc. It was her blood that did her in. The lady did not have a platelet left. . . ."

What Is Idiopathic Thrombocytopenic Purpura?

It turned out that Bea had died from an autoimmune condition known as *idiopathic thrombocytopenic purpura* (ITP), which occurs when antibodies are directed against blood platelets. Platelets are actually fragments of a large cell called a *megakaryocyte*, which at some point in its life, just cracks like a plate of glass, and becomes fragmented. There are hundreds of megakaryocytes in the blood and thousands of platelets that come from one fragmented cell. When someone has ITP, the antiplatelet antibodies bind to the surface of platelets as if they were antigens. As these immune complexes circulate together in the bloodstream, the spleen sees them as abnormal and removes them from circulation. The more platelets are removed, the lower the level of platelets left in the blood. Because platelets are responsible for clotting, a lower platelet count makes hemorrhaging more likely. A normal platelet count is around 130,000 platelets per cubic millimeter. People whose platelets drop into the 30,000 to 50,000 range can hemorrhage even after a very small cut, or, when the skin is not broken, the blood will pool under the skin, resulting in a bruise or a hematoma. If the platelets fall below 15,000, there can be spontaneous bleeding even in instances where there is no injury. Bea's platelet count was virtually zero, because she had ignored all of the signs of platelet absence for such a protracted period of time.

An easy way to understand idiopathic thrombocytopenic purpura is to break down its name into the component parts. Idiopathic means that no one really understands what causes the disease. Thrombocytopenic means that the disease is related to low levels of thrombocytes, which is another name for platelets. Purpura refers to the purple or red raised patches that are generated by bleeding from the capillaries just under the skin.

Curious and, I admit it, a bit embarrassed, later that day I called the police and got the background on the woman. The police had earlier spoken with Bea's husband, who had flown in from Japan and landed at midnight. Shocked and distraught, he filled in the story as best he could, with an amazing memory for detail, particularly under the circumstances.

It seems that several years ago, Bea had casually remarked to her husband that her gums had started bleeding and that her menstrual periods were extending far beyond her usual five days. But it was not until she noticed a series of bruises on her legs, arms, and breasts that she thought to see Dr. T., her internist. The bruises prompted an instant response from Dr. T. who, on seeing them, ordered an immediate blood test and platelet count. Her platelet count came back dangerously below normal, and the doctor told her that this was a serious situation. He suggested more comprehensive studies to explain this astonishing loss of platelets, one of which would be a bone marrow biopsy. Bea refused, calling the test "too scary." He then suggested clotting studies of platelet activity, which she refused again, citing the expense. In retrospect, her husband said, she may have been frightened of the results, distrusting of the doctor, or actually reluctant to spend the money, which was tight because the two had planned to start a family in the near future.

Because she was not feeling sick, she decided to take matters into her own hands and to try to cure herself with alternative medicine. Before moving to the suburbs, Bea had lived in Greenwich Village and still had a number of friends there. One of these friends knew of a man who sold Chinese herbs. The friend swore by the man, who she said had helped another friend with her sciatica. So it was not long after that conversation that Dr. T., a graduate of Tufts Medical School and trained at The Peter Bent Brigham Hospital in Boston, was replaced by Mr. Qui of Chinatown, purveyor of the finest in Oriental herbs and alternative medicines this side of Mott Street. (See chapter 20 for a discussion of medicinal herbs.)

Initially, Mr. Qui sold Bea a series of powders consisting of a variety of plant extracts and one particular root obtained from a tree in the southern part of China. He explained that they were a panacea for all kinds of immune diseases and conditions of overactive bodily functions. He also sold her a brown bag full of "gumballs," pills that he assured her would fill her with energy. Indeed, not long after ingesting some twelve "gumball" pills and six capsules per day of tree roots downed with herb tea, Bea felt better and the bruises went away. Eventually, she discontinued all of her herbal treatment and remained symptom-free for several months. Then the bruising returned. At that point she simply went on the same alternative regimen as before, never returning to her physician and only visiting Mr. Qui once more for a "gumball" refill.

On the night in question she had just returned from a three-day visit to her sister at the Jersey Shore, which was planned to coincide with her husband's business trip to Japan. The stay was uneventful, except that the day before Bea was supposed to return home she developed a sore throat, a slight fever, and joint pains. Her sister gave her some aspirin and made Bea promise to see a "real" doctor the next day. According to Bea's husband, who spoke to her just before boarding the airplane for New Jersey, she complained of feeling "lousy," as though a truck had hit her. She was going to take a bath and get into bed, she said, and would see him when he got home. That was just about an hour before her neighbor found Bea on the bathroom floor.

Many young women die each year from ITP either because their doctors do not recognize the disease, because they themselves do not pay attention to the signs and symptoms of the illness, or, as in Bea's case, because they do not follow medical advice. You cannot ignore low platelets. It is a mistake that will surely come back to haunt you. I earlier mentioned that platelets are essential to the clotting of blood. When the platelets are very low, or, as in Bea's case almost nonexistent, a person can bleed to death in a matter of minutes.

Here is what I believe happened to Bea. She drove home from the shore feeling poorly. The infection she had developed days before probably set off her immune system, and things started heading in a downward spiral. Her already low platelets dropped further, which is what a viral infection will do to someone who already has compromised platelets. She probably came home, dressed for bed, and went into the bathroom. When she was on the toilet she must have strained while pushing, ruptured a vessel in her brain and bled into her head. This is called a Valsalva maneuver. Unfortunately, it is not an uncommon cause of death, particularly in people with high blood pressure.

In keeping with the mechanisms of ITP, the pinpoint petechiae marks in her eyes and on her face and cheeks were the result of small capillaries hemorrhaging as she strained. She also hemorrhaged around her eyes and her rectum. The bruising around her rectum was probably the result of Bea cleaning herself after going to the toilet earlier that day. Finally, the marks around her neck were marks she sustained when the paramedic placed the endotracheal tube in her windpipe to help her breathe. His slight degree of pressure on her neck while tilting back her head so he could see the opening of her trachea was enough to cause bruising in someone who had no platelets.

True, Bea was not murdered. But her death was completely unnecessary. One could cast blame in many directions in this case, but the real individual to blame is the victim herself. Bea ignored the pleas of her physician and the reality of her disease.

Let us talk first about the issue of alternative medicine. I have a problem with patients who partake of alternative medicine when they do so instead of taking prescribed medications, especially in the face of a life-threatening condition. In Bea's case, she denied the seriousness of her disease and was duped into thinking that the naturopathic drugs were treating her condition. I use the term "duped" because the contents of the drugs or herbs she was sold were not listed any-where, so she could not have known what she was ingesting. The gumballs—if they were anything like the ones I have seen from simi-lar health and herb establishments—probably contained enough ste-roids to make her feel good, as steroids will do, and so she thought she was controlling her disease. As far as I am concerned, if the man-ufacturers were known, and they are usually not known, they should be prosecuted.

Then there is the issue of her doctor. Should he have pressed his pa-tient harder to submit to the tests he suggested? Did he have the right to call her husband to inform him of the serious nature of her condi-tion? In retrospect, of course he did, but in this litigious society that defends patients' rights above all others, it is not surprising that he did not act. This is not a unique situation by any means. In these days of time-measured office visits, who among us has time to go chasing down a missing patient?

The immune system is not to be toyed with, and often the dangers can be silent, as they were in Bea's case. The destruction of platelets can happen through a variety of mechanisms. Platelets can be im-peded early on in the bone marrow. Destruction of the platelet mother cell is common with chemical poisoning, which could be from chemotherapy, but also from exposure to petroleum, ether, ben-zene, or many other toxic chemicals in the environment. Drugs also can cause platelet destruction, especially quinine or sulfa drugs. The most common cause of low platelets, however, is accelerated destruc-tion, which is strictly an immune mechanism. The immune process of demolishing platelets can result from leukemia or lymphoma and can be associated with lupus or Sjögren's syndrome.

Treating ITP

When it is recognized early, ITP is easy to treat. When the platelets are dangerously low, patients are generally prescribed corticosteroids, such as prednisone, to slow down the immune response. As you may remember, it was steroids that more than likely were in the gumballs that Bea took, which may account for why she felt better so fast and continued to feel well for a while.

If the ITP does not respond to prednisone, I give patients pooled immunoglobulin (IVIG). These pooled antibodies are taken from blood donors, purified, and infused into a patient with low platelets to elevate the platelet level. This treatment, which is safe and effective (and very expensive), cannot cure the disease, however, nor can it sustain the elevated platelet levels indefinitely.

If the platelets continue to drop, the next step is to remove the spleen. Recall from chapter 1 that the spleen is the repository where the immune system takes unwanted debris that results from destruction of antigens. It is also the dumping ground for our old red and white cells, and our major filter for diseased materials. Accordingly, the spleen acts like a filter that can sequester the platelets if they are part of an immune complex, and such platelets are trapped and not available to help the blood clot. With the spleen gone, the platelets can continue to circulate in the bloodstream and help with clotting.

Removal of the spleen is not my first choice for ITP or any immune disorder in which there are low platelets. If it becomes necessary, though, I will do it because I believe the pros outweigh the cons. For example, patients with no spleen are more susceptible to bacterial infections, particularly the various types of pneumonia. This is why I give anyone with a removed spleen a flu vaccine and Pneumovax, the vaccine for pneumonia.

A final treatment for ITP, which can be done before or after removing the spleen, is called platelet infusion. This procedure calls for the transfusion of someone else's platelets into the patient with autoimmune disease. I do not use this treatment if I can avoid it because if the patient already has an antibody against his or her own platelets, a transfusion might bring into the body another antigen on somebody else's platelets, which would ultimately leave that patient to make new antibodies against a completely new antigen.

When I think of Bea, I regret that she did not live long enough to read this chapter, although I am not sure even this explanation would have been convincing enough. The will can be an insurmountable opponent. This case is the exception and not the rule, I might add, because people rarely bleed to death from ITP as Bea did. They usually get medical help when things start to go noticeably wrong. For me, the case was remarkable in so many respects, but mostly because it is so unusual to see a case of ITP on an emergency call. The disease is so easy to treat that it rarely gets to the point that it causes massive bleeding in a crisis situation. Also, it is so rare that my EMS life crosses paths with my immunologic life. With all due respect to this poor woman, for me to be on call and have the "villain" turn out to be autoimmune disease was nothing short of amazing.

CHAPTER FIVE

TYPE 1 JUVENILE DIABETES

When Sweetness Falls from Grace

LIKE ANY OTHER eleven-year-old girl, Elizabeth spent her day at school and at play, with family and with friends. The daughter of a prominent New York politician and his wife, she seemed to be living a normal, happy life. Then one day, her mother noticed that she was behaving most unusually. She was drinking quarts, not glasses, of water to quench her thirst—and she did this quite often. Understandably, she began making frequent trips to the bathroom, sometimes many in a single hour. Within weeks, the attractive and social young girl suddenly developed a ravenous appetite, totally unlike to her normal eating habits. What was of more concern to her parents was the fact that despite the huge amounts of food she consumed, Elizabeth was always hungry, and, despite it all, she was losing weight.

By now terribly worried, Elizabeth's parents took their daughter to see the family doctor, who immediately referred them to see Dr. F. M. Allen, who ran the Physiatric Institute in Morristown, New Jersey. Doctor Allen was a specialist in children's diabetes and had written many books, including a definitive account of the disease. His treatment methods at the clinic, while highly controversial, seemed to work. By using his technique, he had successfully managed the diabetes in many youngsters in Elizabeth's situation. Much like Mr. Bumble in *Oliver Twist*, Dr. Allen boarded these waif-like children, and then he severely limited their food.

When Elizabeth and her parents arrived in Morristown, Dr. Allen examined her and explained to her parents that the child, who now weighed seventy-five pounds, unquestionably had diabetes, a disease in which the body can no longer process food and turn it into the fuel it requires. He admitted Elizabeth to his clinic that day and immediately put her on a strict diet of between 400 and 600 calories a day, taken from lean meat, eggs, milk, vegetables, and a little fruit. She ate like this six days a week, and the seventh day she fasted. Her parents sent a nurse to attend her at the clinic during her stay and the nurse was with her continuously, in part to make sure Elizabeth did not deviate from the sparse and regimented diet. After three months at the clinic, a weak and very frail young Elizabeth, now thinner than ever, returned home with her nurse, and for the next three years, difficult as it was, she managed to subsist on Dr. Allen's semi-starvation diet. If her parents were sometimes distraught at the effect of this diet on their daughter, now fourteen, they had only to recall that at that time there were no long-term survivors of childhood diabetes. The year was 1921.

Two major events that occurred that year made a great mark on Elizabeth's family. In the first, her father, Charles Hughes, was named U.S. Secretary of State (he was later, from 1930 to 1941, Chief Justice of the Supreme Court). The second event, however, would have a far greater impact on people around the world. That year, two young men, one a physician only five years out of medical school and the other a medical student, were busily at work in a small laboratory on the campus of the University of Toronto, trying to find a way to treat the glucose excess in the blood of diabetic patients. At the time, doctors already knew that the pancreas was connected to the regulation of blood sugar, but no one quite knew how to use this information for treatment. Dr. Fredrick Banting and his assistant Charles Best thought they knew. They spent the summer taking pancreatic tissue from dogs or calf fetuses and pulverizing it into a solution. After finally perfecting the chemistry of this solution, on July 10, 1921, the two young scientists injected their perfected extract solution into a dog whose pancreas had earlier been removed to render it diabetic. The dog's glucose level decreased from 50 percent above normal to normal in less than an hour. The men had discovered insulin.

In February 1922, Banting and Best published their work, *The Internal Secretion of the Pancreas*, and the whole world, including Charles Hughes, learned of the breakthrough. In August, after much correspondence with the two noted men, Mrs. Hughes brought Elizabeth to Toronto. There, the emaciated child, almost fifteen years old and weighing only forty-five pounds, began receiving insulin daily from Dr. Banting. She was able to eat again, whatever she wanted, as much as she wanted—including the earlier forbidden carbohydrates. Within three months, Elizabeth and her nurse came home to Washington. At that point she consumed up to 2,200 calories a day. Two months later, she weighed a normal 110 pounds.

What Is Type 1 Diabetes?

As Elizabeth's story illustrates, diabetes is a chronic condition characterized by high blood sugar levels. Blood sugar levels are normally regulated by insulin, which is manufactured by the pancreas. Diabetes transpires when the pancreas does not produce sufficient insulin, or the cells do not respond to it.

There are three different types of diabetes, only one of which—type 1—is autoimmune. Before discussing type 1 in depth, I want to point up the differences among three types of diabetes.

▷ *Type 1 (autoimmune) diabetes*, the subject of this chapter, is formally called insulin-dependent diabetes mellitus (IDDM) and is also known as juvenile diabetes, although it can begin in adulthood. Autoimmune diabetes occurs when the immune system looks upon the insulin-producing cells of the pancreas as foreign and attacks them, inflaming the pancreatic tissue and robbing the pancreas of its ability to produce insulin. Once this process has begun, the pancreas is eventually rendered useless.

▷ *Type II diabetes*, which is a completely different disease than type 1, is far more common and usually affects adults over forty. This disease is not autoimmune-related. People with type II diabetes produce insulin, but their bodies do not use it efficiently. In such cases, blood sugar is kept under control with medication, diet, and exercise. If these therapies do not work well enough, insulin injections become necessary.

▷ *Gestational diabetes*, which also is not autoimmune-related, is a metabolic condition that affects some pregnant women, generally in midpregnancy, and goes away when the baby is born. While we do not know for sure why this occurs during pregnancy, we do know that it results from the body's resistance to insulin. Gestational diabetes is usually treated with diet and exercise.

The Diabetes Process

When we eat, our food is broken down into proteins, fats, and simple sugars from carbohydrates. The liver processes these nutrients into glucose, a type of sugar that is the main source of energy for all cells in the body, something akin to putting gasoline in a car. Glucose molecules float in the bloodstream waiting to be called upon to enter the cells, but they can only enter the cells in the presence of the hormone insulin, which stands like a sentry at the door. Insulin is a protein that is composed of amino acids. If there is no insulin to "open" the cell, the glucose cannot pass through. A glucose-starved cell leads to many serious repercussions in the body. For example, as an organ is deprived of energy, it has to work that much harder to keep things running. This is why untreated diabetics lack energy and are so tired all the time. Also, if there is no insulin to push sugar into the cells, the glucose has nowhere to go and eventually builds up in the bloodstream, yielding a potentially dangerous condition known as *high blood sugar*.

When there is a buildup of sugar in the blood, the kidneys go to work producing extra urine to try to excrete it. To provide enough urine to rid the body of the excess glucose, sometimes the kidney must extract water from the tissues. When that occurs, the tissues become dehydrated, which is why untreated diabetics are excessively thirsty and drink a lot, a condition known as *polydipsia*. Moreover, it is no surprise that by drinking an excessive amount of liquid, the diabetic will follow with frequent urination, or *polyuria*. When the cells lack glucose, they begin to burn fat and eventually call on the body's supply of protein, which leads to the diabetic's need to replenish protein, a situation that manifests itself in excessive eating, or *polyphagia*, without feeling full.

Also, when there is no glucose for energy, the cells may look elsewhere for alternative fuel. In many cases they turn to the liver, which, in its efforts to help out, produces acidic substances called *ketones*. If too many ketones are produced and not used, they accumulate in the blood, lowering the overall pH of the blood and making it abnormally acidic. This extra acidity creates a potentially life-threatening situation called *ketoacidosis*, which can affect the electrical conduction of the heart and severely depress the nervous system. Symptoms of ketoacidosis include abdominal pain, vomiting, rapid breathing, extreme tiredness, and drowsiness. If diabetes persists, the walls of the blood vessels, most notably the capillaries, may also be damaged, compromising the blood supply to the kidneys, eyes, and the limbs, and ultimately placing these essential body parts in jeopardy.

It is amazing to think that all this can be alleviated with a small amount of insulin.

Causes of Diabetes

As with so many of the other autoimmune diseases, we do not know why the immune system attacks and destroys certain cells—in this case insulin-producing cells. There may be a combination of factors, ranging from viral to hereditary. Viruses such as mumps, German measles, and Coxsackie virus B are known to attack the pancreas. It has also recently been reported that enteroviral diarrhea-producing viruses are two times more common in children who developed diabetes than in their siblings. We know now that diabetic children are more likely to be born to mothers who have antibodies against this virus in their blood. There are probably many other infectious causes that lead to alteration of the cell surface, making it look like an antigen so that the immune system comes in and destroys it.

As for the hereditary factors, there are many clues to the origin of this debilitating disease but no specific culprit that we can put a finger on—not yet, anyway. We do know that certain genes on chromosome 6, where all the immune response genes are located, can make one genetically susceptible to diabetes. Just how the genetic component works has not been scientifically established, but some believe that it has to do with T-cell receptors. In other words, one must have a T-cell receptor with exactly the right fit that allows it to attach to an antigen. Only then can there be an immune complex that will ultimately invade and destroy the pancreas.

Some unconventional but rather creative experiments show that antibodies to cow's milk protein can cross-react with the receptor on the islet cells that regulate the release of insulin. In other words, a few researchers suspect that drinking milk at a young age might predispose one to immune-mediated diabetes. This theory has met with much controversy but I mention it here because it is currently the subject of study.

Nancy's Story

According to recent statistics reported by the National Institutes of Health in 2001, at least 1 million Americans have type 1 diabetes. Each year, between 11,000 and 12,000 children are newly diagnosed. My patient, Nancy, was one of those children. I would like to share her story because her experience is prototypical of a young child facing this disease.

I first met Nancy several years ago, when she was nine years old. Her parents, owners of a small dry cleaning business, brought her to my office. Nancy is small for her age, but not frail, by any means. She has a face full of freckles, big brown eyes, and an infectious smile. She looks exactly like her father. I learned within the first several minutes of her visit that from the time she was six, her life has revolved around ice skating. Her parents told me that according to her coaches, Nancy had "the gift" that turns ordinary skaters into

Olympic stars. "This is why we work so hard to ensure her ice time, lessons, and equipment," her father said.

After the four of us talked for a while, I asked Nancy to tell me about a typical day for her. She explained, in the animated style of a nine-year-old, that her day normally began with one parent dropping her off at skating practice at 6 A.M. At eight o'clock, she would exchange her skates for sneakers, and one of her parents would drive her from the rink to school. Sometimes, if there was a competition coming up, she would stay at the rink an extra hour for a lesson. Her father interjected that this was done with the sanction of the school because her teachers—those who had seen her skate—agreed that Nancy was, indeed, a very talented young girl.

When I asked them to describe the experience that brought them to me, Nancy's mother spoke first: "I'm not sure when it started," she said. "I suppose I should have seen that there was something physically wrong. Several weeks ago, Nancy began to look a bit lethargic at home. But I shrugged it off to tiredness from skating combined with school. She's a very diligent student and never goes to sleep without finishing her homework."

At that point, Nancy's father added: "We noticed she seemed to be losing weight and so we kept pushing her to eat a little bit more, which she did, but she kept getting thinner. My wife planned to take her for a checkup as soon as the competition was over. But one thing always leads to another—you know how these things are—it seems there was always another competition." He described a morning, one of those late mornings, when she skated late. He had dropped her off and gone directly to work. When he arrived at his store, he learned from a helper that Nancy was being taken by ambulance to the local hospital.

The way her teacher described it later, Nancy had walked into the classroom, literally shuffled to her desk, put down her head and fell asleep. Nancy's classmate, Bordon, called to the teacher that something was wrong with Nancy and that she smelled funny. The teacher approached the child and noted a strong smell of what she thought was alcohol, if somewhat sweeter. When the teacher could not arouse Nancy, she sent Bordon running to the principal's office to summon the school nurse, who called an ambulance.

By the time Nancy arrived at the hospital, she was in a coma with potentially lethal high blood sugar—a condition known as diabetic ketoacidosis (DKA). While a very high level of blood sugar is an integral part this condition, it is not the only aspect. Diabetes-associated dehydration and severe derangement of minerals in the body also can be quite lethal. Because there was so little insulin to push the sugar in her blood into the cells of her muscles and organs, Nancy was left with high levels of toxic chemicals—*acetoacetate* and *beta hydroxybutyrate*—in her blood. These chemicals caused the DKA and ultimately, the sweet alcohol smell she emitted.

In the ambulance, Nancy received fluids intravenously to reverse the dehydration, insulin to push the sugar into her cells, and potassium and bicarbonates to change the acidity of her blood and provide enough vital minerals to allow her heart and other vital organs to stabilize. Had it remained untreated, the DKA could have had severe physical consequences. Instead, the hydration and insulin therapy brought her around within an hour and when she awoke, she reported feeling better than she had in weeks.

Treating Diabetes

Nancy's parents were heartbroken to learn their daughter had diabetes, but I quickly assured them that this need not interfere with her skating. She could go on to become a champion, *if* she took care of herself. At first it would take some doing on everyone's part, but it was not that difficult once the commitment was made. After all, there are around 100,000 children in this country living with this condition and their lives, with some modifications, are quite normal.

"I don't know your daughter all that well, but she seems to be an extremely disciplined child," I told them. "I have no reason to believe she can't just weave her self-care into her daily life and, with a few modifications, return to skating as well." This brought smiles of relief all around.

Children and adults with diabetes can live an essentially normal life, but they clearly must modify their lifestyles. While it may seem daunting at first, eventually each step becomes just another part of the day. I assured Nancy's parents that her condition was quite manageable. I then outlined for them what I felt her major needs would be.

I started by explaining that people with diabetes need to keep blood, exercise, and insulin in balance in order to control blood sugar levels. When the balance is disturbed, the child will face problems. For example, if her blood sugar falls below normal, a situation referred to as *hypoglycemia*, she may feel lethargic, cranky, hungry, and weak. If it gets too low, she may lose consciousness or lapse into a coma. This situation can be treated immediately by eating or drinking something that contains sugar. I suggested that Nancy's coach should be made aware of her condition so that he could provide a candy bar or juice if it should become necessary. I explained that in diabetes, the opposite also can also occur. *Hyperglycemia* means too much sugar in the blood. This is brought on by overeating, lack of exercise, insufficient insulin, or a combination. Symptoms include extreme thirst, frequent urination, fatigue, weight loss, and vomiting.

Then I laid out the following rules for managing diabetes, which I suggest for all my diabetic patients:

▷ Most important, the child (or parent) will have to carefully monitor her blood sugar (glucose) perhaps several times a day. This has become much easier than in the past when children were required to stick themselves with painful needles and then wait for the results for several minutes. Now, very small devices can measure the blood sugar painlessly and can give an accurate readout in seconds.

▷ Insulin must be taken daily by injection. Injection is the only way to provide insulin, because taking it by mouth would first send it to the stomach, and stomach acid destroys proteins like insulin. Children as young as six can and do inject themselves. But there are now insulin pumps available as well, and some children seem more comfortable with them. These are portable computerized devices that attach to the body and administer continuous, small amounts of insulin over the course of the day.

▷ It is essential, early on, to keep a diary of blood sugar measurements. This information can help a doctor establish patterns of activity and food consumption and evaluate their effects on insulin levels.

▷ Diet is crucial. While each person is different and should be prescribed for by her own doctor, most doctors suggest that a certain percentage of the diet come from carbohydrates (50–60 percent), protein (20–25 percent), and fats (20–30 percent). Most diets are consumed in a meal/snack pattern, and it is advised to eat six times a day.

▷ Regular exercise is essential because it helps control blood sugar and burn calories, thus keeping the weight at an optimal level.

▷ Because diabetes compromises circulation, it is important to take particular care of the feet and to examine them for small cuts, blisters, or sores that may not heal easily.

▷ Because the immune system is not the same in a diabetic as it is in a nondiabetic, diabetics are more susceptible to infection, and if an infection occurs, it has to be cared for more aggressively.

Nancy's parents were concerned about what would happen if, for some reason, she missed a dose of insulin. I explained that if that occurred, she'd get tired and lose strength, perhaps. But her diabetes wouldn't go out of control to the point that she would suffer serious complications from one or two missed shots. It is only after many years of being out of control that severe complications occur.

Nancy will need to come back to see me periodically to measure her hemoglobin A_{1C}, a test to tell us whether the diabetes is under control. It reflects the amount of red blood cells that are connected to sugar.

Complications of Uncontrolled Diabetes

The importance of keeping diabetes under control is nowhere so well illustrated as in a discussion of the complications that can occur from neglect. Following are some of the more common diabetic complications:

Nerve damage. Peripheral neuropathy—damage to nerves in the feet, legs, and hands—leads to lack of sensation in these areas. Numbness of the feet in particular can lead to unfelt injuries. If you cannot feel a sore or small injury, the tendency is to neglect it. When circulation is poor, as happens with diabetes, the tissue heals very slowly, if at all. The more compromised the circulation, the harder it is to heal a wound or skin ulcer. Ultimately, unhealed wounds can break down and the only way to treat them is by amputation. This is far more often a problem in adults than in children.

Eye problems. When circulation is compromised, the retina of the eye can be affected. This means the rods and cones portion of the eye or that which discerns color and shapes can be damaged. In some serious cases, blindness can result.

Kidney damage. If the blood vessels to the kidney are affected in an adverse way, the filtering mechanisms of the kidney can shut down, with the result that protein leaks into the urine. Untreated kidney problems can lead to kidney failure, which means that toxic materials, instead of being excreted, build up in the blood.

Atherosclerosis. This refers to a buildup of plaque on the inside walls of the blood vessels. Depending on the location of the plaque, such a buildup can lead to serious complications such as stroke and heart disease.

Pregnancy and Diabetes

Today women with diabetes can expect to have healthy babies, but of course there are risks. I strongly advise all my patients of child-bearing age to plan their pregnancies rather than just let nature take its course.

If the mother-to-be has diabetes, the pregnancy is high risk, no question. For example, several recent studies have linked abnormal hemoglobin A_{1C} values during early pregnancy to an increase of spontaneous abortion and congenital abnormalities. The hemoglobin A_{1C} (HgA_{1C}) test measures the caramelization (yes, just like chewy sugar candies) of the hemoglobin (red pigment) in the blood. If the blood sugar is very high for some time, the HgA_{1C} or sugar coated hemoglobin will be very high, indicating that blood sugar is not well controlled. In another test, 13 percent of babies born to diabetic mothers have abnormal hemoglobin A_{1C} values compared with 2 percent of babies born to nondiabetic mothers.

Women and their physicians need to do whatever they can to minimize the risk of premature and late fetal loss or hereditary abnormalities to the child. Unfortunately, most problems in the fetus occur within the first seven weeks of the pregnancy, a time when many women do not even know that they are pregnant. Therefore, pregnancy planning is very important. Women should not plan a pregnancy if their kidneys are failing, if they are losing an uncomfortable amount of weight, or if they are *ketoacidotic.*

Prepregnancy counseling must be a part of every diabetic woman's plan. Considering the health of the mother is as important as that of the baby. Diabetes can worsen during pregnancy, and a woman can have low sugar levels with ketoacidosis. Blood vessel disease can get worse, infections can ravage the kidneys, and among other things, the mother can go into preterm labor. If the mother-to-be has normal or close to normal blood glucose levels before her pregnancy and then into the early stages of the pregnancy, she should have a healthy baby.

Some Final Thoughts on Diabetes

The only way to cure diabetes is to replace the nonfunctioning pancreas with a pancreatic transplant or transplant of the pancreatic islet cells. Progress has its price, however, and the cost of such a transplant is far more than financial. One drawback is the difficulty in finding a suitable pancreas, but beyond that, the procedure requires that the patient take powerful antirejection drugs. In a person with an already compromised immune system, this is not always a good idea. Still, many diabetics have had successful pancreas transplants, and a number have islet cell transplants. The islet cells are really the workhorse of the pancreas, because these cells make the insulin that keeps blood sugar at normal range. Currently, researchers are working on a way to encapsulate islet cells in semipermeable membrane "packages" that would protect them from attack by the immune system but allow insulin to be secreted. For now, it appears that if surgery is done, whole pancreas transplantation is the more common way of getting the islet cells into the individual with diabetes.

Would encapsulated islet-cell transplants have seemed like science fiction to Elizabeth Hughes? Probably not. In fact, toward the end of her life—and it was a long one—she probably was familiar with most of this research and actually lived long enough to read about it. This young girl who might have died—but for the good luck to be alive at the right time—ultimately received a degree from Barnard College. In 1930, she married William Gosset, a lawyer who later became a vice president of the Ford Motor Company. In 1981, after an active life filled with family and friends—and after spending fifty-eight years on insulin—Elizabeth Hughes Gosset died of a heart attack at the age of seventy-three. During her lifetime, very few people knew about her diabetes.

CHAPTER SIX

MULTIPLE SCLEROSIS

Electricity without Insulation

---

*I*n medicine, it sometimes turns out that the most anguishing, bizarre, or difficult cases are the ones that stay with you forever. "I'll never forget that heart," you might say, if you were a cardiac surgeon. "Six bypasses! Imagine!" But other times it is the patients themselves whom you never forget, simply because the people who had those diseases were so special to you. Long after their disease disappears from your mind, those people are still there. I have been lucky and had many such patients. There were four in a year once—four women who actually came to see me within the span of three months. All four had the same condition and all were about the same age, early to mid-thirties. Their stories, however, were and continue to be markedly different:

Ann is thirty-six and a senior editor at a book publishing company. She is being honored at a beautiful luncheon with her publisher's award for excellence. She strides to the stage to accept the honor, politely thanks the woman who introduced her, lays out her speech on the lectern, and attempts to read. But what she sees instead of a speech is a red-green blur—nothing else. Despite a sudden dull ache in her right eye, she charmingly ad-libs what she remembers from the speech, and no one is any the wiser.

On another end of town, Cynthia passes the same coffee table in her living room three times in as many days and bumps her shin each time. She slams her elbow on the kitchen sink two days later in an effort to catch her balance. That weekend, as she leaves the shower, her husband sees her bruises and jokingly asks who has been beating her up.

Jane walks home from the park for lunch pushing her two children in their stroller and suddenly finds she is too weak to go another block. Overcome by heat, she sits down on a nearby bench and calls a friend to come and rescue her. While she waits, she silently thanks whoever it was that invented the cell phone. Her friend picks her up ten minutes later.

Sarah has just graduated at the top of her law-school class. It all came easy to her and now, after studying for four weeks, she has no worries whatsoever about the New York Bar Exam. The day arrives, she goes into Room 106 to take the test, looks at the questions, and is stunned to find she cannot remember some of what she knew "cold" the day before. (She passed anyway.)

You are quite correct in wondering what these four women in different corners of a single city might have in common. They were each encountering, in distinct ways, the first evidence of multiple sclerosis (MS). Although MS is often a multisymptom disease, early in the course of events only a single symptom is present, and as you have seen above, no two people exhibit their manifestations in precisely the same way.

What Is Multiple Sclerosis?

Multiple sclerosis is a disorder of the brain and spinal cord, which together comprise the central nervous system (CNS). Symptoms of MS, only some of which you read about above, are caused by progressive damage to the outer covering of nerve cells, called the *myelin sheath.* The myelin sheath is a fatty covering that insulates the bundle of nerves, similar to the thin rubber coating on a telephone wire. The disease begins when an overly aggressive group of T cells mistakenly think the covering of the nerve cells are antigens and eat their way through the protective sheath, leaving patches of inflamed tissue, called plaques, in their wake.

This process of stripping myelin or insulation from the nerves is called *demyelination.* When demyelination occurs, the nerves within the sheath are disturbed, leading to an interruption or complete blocking of impulses to nerves in distant body regions. The blocked impulses cause a breakdown in communication between components of the central nervous system and the specific areas of the body that are governed by it. The outcome is that the brain cannot instruct the body on how to balance, move, feel, or, on rare occasions, even think.

There are three kinds of MS: *relapsing/remitting* (more often now called simply remitting), *progressive,* and *benign. Remitting* MS is the most common type and is characterized by at least two attacks of any severity or duration, interrupted by a period of remission during which there are no symptoms whatsoever. Remission occurs when the inflammation subsides and the neurons resume their proper function. Remission also can occur because the brain has *plasticity*, that is, it has the ability to change and even regrow. Plasticity of the brain is a marvelous capability when you consider that even if a stroke or some physical injury brings brain function to a temporary halt, the brain itself has an extraordinary resilience—a healing process that can sometimes return it to normal, depending, of course, on how much damage has been done. Accordingly, if the need should arise following the onset of MS, new neuronal pathways (like strings of electrical wiring that conduct messages throughout the body) and connections can form their own bypasses around the damaged neurons.

Progressive MS generally starts slowly and evolves into a more gradual development of symptoms that simply get worse over a period of months or years. *Benign* MS is described as the type that occurs when the patient suffers only one or two mild exacerbations and no permanent disability.

Causes and Demographics

No one knows what causes MS. Like so many other autoimmune diseases, it is thought to be part genetic and part environmental. Although there is not yet a named gene that causes MS, some researchers believe it is likely that MS may have some hereditary factors. This is because in identical twins, the chance that the second twin will develop MS if the first has it is 30 percent, whereas in fraternal twins the number is 4 percent. We also know that 10 percent of patients with MS will have an affected family member.

Viruses have been linked to MS as a cause since the disease was first described. Viruses such as herpes, measles, Epstein-Barr, and an assortment of nonviruses such as chlamydia all have been implicated at one time or another. None of these has been proven the cause, however. Precisely which virus is involved is not known, but we are looking for it.

Demographic statistics recently issued lead us to believe that MS may be induced genetically, environmentally, and hormonally. For example:

▷ Whites are more than twice as likely as other races to develop MS, while the Inuit Eskimos and Gypsies never get MS.
▷ MS is thought to be five times more prevalent in the northern United States, Canada, and Europe than in the tropical regions, although this has never been entirely proven.
▷ Women of European and Scandinavian populations get MS, but it is generally not found in Asians, Africans, or native Indians of North and South America.
▷ African-American women have a higher rate of MS than women who live in Africa, which supports the theory that environment has something to do with MS risk. And, as mentioned above, MS is five times more prevalent in the northern United States, Canada, and Europe than in the tropical regions.

The NIH estimates that approximately 250,000 to 350,000 people in the United States have been diagnosed with MS. The condition attacks adults primarily between the ages of twenty and forty. Rarely are new cases diagnosed in people younger than fifteen or older than sixty. While in the progressive form of MS, the sex ratio between men and women is equal, in the far more common relapsing/remitting form, 70 to 75 percent of patients are women. This probably has something to do with hormonal influences, but there are no supporting data as yet. Personally, I believe the way MS behaves in pregnant women upholds this theory.

Symptoms of Multiple Sclerosis

As was illustrated in our four earlier examples, symptoms of MS can be wide ranging. Duration and magnitude of symptoms also may vary. Because nerves are everywhere throughout the body, MS-related symptoms can and do show up just about anywhere. Specific symptoms of MS depend on where in the central nervous system the demyelination takes place and which body part is on the receiving end of the neuronal messages. Lesions can be found anywhere in the white matter of the central nervous system, including the cerebral hemispheres of the brain (motor activity), the optic nerve (vision), the brain stem (breathing and heart rate), and the cerebellum (coordination and athletic ability.) The white matter of the spinal cord also serves specific areas of the body. For example, if demyelination occurs near the nerves that serve the bladder, then the bladder is affected. Or if they are near the perineum or the pudendum (the nerves to the pubic area), this leads to erectile dysfunction or spastic bladder. Other corticospinal tract lesions cause the muscular weakness and the spasticity of the lower extremities.

On a more personal level, my four patients perfectly illustrate the variety of symptoms that can befall people with MS. Anne, for example, experienced one of the more common first symptoms of MS— blurred vision and red-green color distortion. People with eye manifestations will sometimes experience pain or transient blindness in one eye. (For some unknown reason, eye problems generally subside in the later stages of MS.) Her eye pain most likely stemmed from a condition called *optic neuritis*, or put more simply, inflammation of the optic nerve. Double vision, another characteristic symptom, is the result of a slightly paralyzed eye muscle.

Cynthia lost her balance due to muscle weakness and lack of coordination, which most MS patients experience in their extremities at some point over the course of the illness. At the much later stages, these symptoms can impair walking or standing. Conversely, rather than experiencing weakness, some people have spasticity, or increased muscle tone, leading to stiffness and spasms. A patient can have spasticity and weakness at different times, but these symptoms can also occur simultaneously.

Sarah drew a blank on her law boards, but it is actually rare to suffer an acute memory lapse so early in the game. Still, it is estimated that up to 50 percent of people with MS experience some cognitive difficulties such as poor concentration, lack of memory, and difficulty in paying attention, but because the symptoms are so mild most patients are unaware of it. Just to be clear, MS patients do not get dementia—ever. MS patients who are affected by memory lapses cannot remember where they put their glasses or their keys. That is about the extent of it—an exaggerated "senior moment."

Unrelenting fatigue, as it came upon Jane, is by far the most debilitating and chronic symptom of MS. This type of exhaustion may be triggered by physical exertion and subsequently improve with rest, or it may be constant. Because fatigue is such an underlying characteristic, I think it is important to understand, to the degree that it is understandable, the mechanics behind it.

There are many different hypotheses regarding fatigue, but I always think there has to be some common thread that connects patients with autoimmune diseases to this debilitating symptom. Remember from chapters 1 and 2 that cytokines affect everything from the way the ovaries work to the way the brain operates, which includes changing our behavior, to affect sleep and wakefulness, and probably even low-grade fever and fatigue. We know that cytokines float around in the blood supply in the brain. I also believe it's possible that when they are in the brain itself, they actually leave the circulation and act on their own, which is what might cause the extreme fatigue. Many physicians believe this to be the mechanism behind fatigue. I have not found any data yet to support this idea, but I do find it compelling.

Other notable MS symptoms include the following:

▷ Loss of bowel and bladder functions
▷ Constipation of bowel or leakage
▷ Intermittent dizziness
▷ Numbness and tingling of the hands or feet
▷ Joint pain and muscle aches
▷ Sexual dysfunction. This may occur as a result of paresthesias (that is, fleeting feelings of "pins and needles") or a loss of sensation in the pubic area. Women with MS rarely reach orgasm, and most lose their desire to enjoy sex.
▷ Numbness in one leg to the degree that it constantly feels like it is asleep.
▷ Depression. Some form of mental disturbance occurs in over half of patients. I have noted earlier the physical manifestations and cognitive symptoms of MS, but MS can also play a role in changing emotions. Patients have been known to fall victim to severe psychotic disorders, such as manic depression and paranoia. Euphoria and despair, usually seen only in severe cases, also is thought to be due to demyelination of various parts of the brain, including specific areas of the cerebrum and the temporal lobes. (MS also can affect the brain stem, the area of the brain that is responsible for basic functions like breathing.)

Diagnosing Multiple Sclerosis

The unpredictability of MS makes it a difficult disease to diagnose, primarily because it is an episodic disease, which means that MS symptoms are not always present, and when they are, sometimes episodes last only for a few days. Because symptoms must be evident in order for a doctor to make the diagnosis, it is easy to understand why it is so hard. Adding to the difficulty in diagnosing MS is that the symptoms—particularly the early symptoms of fatigue and joint pain—mimic those of a number of other autoimmune disorders, particularly the connective tissue diseases such as lupus, polyarteritis, type 1 diabetes, and Sjögren's syndrome. The difference is that these other autoimmune diseases show involvement beyond the brain and central nervous system, and MS does not.

▷ *History and Physical*

Sometimes, getting to the diagnosis means eliminating other possibilities, which can be a lengthy task. Generally, a neurologist will make the preliminary diagnosis based on the first sign of symptoms. He or she will take a history and do a physical examination. The examination looks for sensory deficits and tests a patient's reflexes and strength. A patient will be asked to walk across the room as the doctor assesses her gait. She may also be given a visual evoked response (VER) test, which looks for vision changes. Both of these symptoms are consistant with early MS.

▷ *Laboratory Tests*

MS is a clinical diagnosis—that is, made by a doctor's observation of signs and symptoms—and generally does not rely on the laboratory. However, as we have just seen, so many diseases can mimic multiple sclerosis that laboratory testing to rule out these other diseases is essential. For example, we will get a Lyme disease test, or look for a viral infection. We also try to rule out inherited illnesses, vitamin deficiencies, and "sticky blood" syndrome (see chapter 3). The only way to eliminate these other possibilities is through negative blood tests. If they are all negative, we start thinking of MS. Sometimes, none of these tests will finalize the diagnosis, and months will go by before we can be sure that a patient has the proper diagnosis. The more tests that are taken, the easier it is to clinch the diagnosis. Here, patience is the key.

▷ *Lumbar Puncture*

Like the lab tests, a lumbar puncture, more commonly known as a spinal tap, is performed more to rule out what is *not* MS than to definitively diagnose what is, but it is still a valuable diagnostic tool.

Certain cellular and chemical abnormalities in the spinal fluid can help define MS. One such chemical is *oligoclonal bands*, which demonstrate that an antibody in the fluid is reacting with the myelin on the nerves. Although oligoclonal bands show up in 95 percent of people who have MS, even this is not definitive because these bands also can be evident in people with *sclerosing panencephalitis* (a rare condition caused by the measles virus) and herpes simplex infections of the brain. The clinical examination and other tests for viral infection can rule these out, however. The mononuclear cell count in the spinal fluid also is helpful in eliminating infections as a cause of symptoms.

▷ *Magnetic Resonance Imaging (MRI)*

I may be dating myself, but I can recall the time before 1977 when there was no MRI, and believe it or not, we thought we were doing just fine, thank you. Not anymore. No MRI? It is positively unthinkable! If you are young enough that you cannot imagine how people existed without cell phones, then you know what I mean. For viewing small areas in great detail, particularly areas of the brain, there is nothing as accurate as the MRI. MRI scanners contain powerful electromagnets that spin around the patient and project the scanned detail on a computer. The images show cross-sections of the area in question, in this case, the brain. They can zoom in on and display even the smallest areas, including the nerves of the brain, and are able to show whether, and to what degree, a nerve is demyelinated—that is, missing insulation. The areas of demyelination show up as white. Upon viewing a demyelinated area within the brain, the neurologist can determine which corresponding area of the body will be affected, and how.

It is important to understand, however, that demyelination by itself does not mean MS is present. You can get a demyelination that looks like MS from other situations that are not autoimmune. For example, a smallpox vaccination, diffuse cerebral sclerosis, encephalomyelitis that follows measles and chickenpox, and even the flu, all can cause lesions that are demyelinating in character, as can rabies and Lyme disease.

▷ *The Hot Bath Test*

Abnormal temperature sensation is a symptom of MS, and nowhere is this better illustrated than when a patient steps into a hot bath or shower. In fact, I have always been amazed to see how quickly MS symptoms are exacerbated by temperature increase (see paragraph below). Sometimes a sensation of weakness comes on so fast that a patient needs help getting out of the tub. Once she is out of the tub or shower and cools off, things become normal again. No one knows why this occurs, but we assume it's because heat increases neurotransmission.

When I was an intern, if we suspected MS in a patient and wanted to determine if we were correct, the patient was asked to take a hot bath. I remember there was only one bathtub on the floor, and all the interns would get together in the late afternoon with our patient. We would take him into to the bathroom at the end of the hall and help him into a very warm tub. Then, we waited for symptoms to occur. As I said, this can happen within seconds, but it also can also take far longer or not occur at all, which is why this test is not done first. Nevertheless, this extraordinary diagnostic test continues to fascinate me to this day.

Treating Multiple Sclerosis

There is no perfect treatment for MS, although recent research into both the immune system and the brain has brought us new therapies. For the most part, these are aimed at slowing the demyelination and mollifying its effects. Because the symptoms of MS are so patient-specific, there are no treatments that can be considered efficacious for everyone.

Immunosuppressives, the hallmark of the treatment for so many other autoimmune diseases, work for patients with MS. But I do not believe they are the best or the most efficient means of dealing with this condition. The problem is that these steroid-type drugs—such as *ACTH* and *methylprednisolone*—have side effects that can render them counterproductive. While steroids can reduce the severity and duration of symptoms in some patients, their side effects with prolonged use include thinning hair, weakened bones, diabetes, accumulation of fat in areas such as the upper back and around the cheeks, and thinning of the skin.

Currently, the most promising new FDA-approved treatments for remitting MS are beta-type interferons. Interferons are cytokines that occur naturally in the human body as a response to viruses. Their role is to regulate the function of the immune system. The synthetic form of interferons is made in the laboratory and used to treat disease. We treat hepatitis C infections and liver disease with beta interferons. Used in the treatment of MS, beta interferons appear to block certain antibodies from attacking the myelin sheaths and may reduce the relapse rate. Treatment can be given weekly, every other week, or three times per week, depending on which one is used. The drug is given by injection either into muscle or under the skin. The type of interferon and the schedule of injection may depend on the type of MS present. The interferons are usually reserved for the relapsing form of MS—the form that comes and goes with no particular regularity—in contrast to the progressive form, in which the patient simply worsens over a long period.

Another new drug, an artificially made polymer called *glatiramer acetate*, is classified as a *tolerance-inducing drug*. This classification of drugs resembles certain antigens and can overpower the immune system's ability to distinguish self from nonself. We use glatiramer acetate to trick the immune system into turning itself off. The drug is also known as a *copaxone* or *copolymer* (a chemical which, when studied in animal models of MS, caused some remission of the disease and, like the interferons, is known to reduce the relapse rate.) The structure of this polymer resembles the myelin basic protein and the strategy is to confuse the immune response. A comparison would be blocking an enemy's radio transmission with a device that causes static. (More on tolerance inducing drugs can be found in chapter 17.)

What You Can Do to Help Yourself

Universally, anyone with MS will do better by following a healthy lifestyle, which means eating a balanced diet of protein, fats, and carbohydrates and getting adequate rest and relaxation to maintain high levels of energy. Avoiding stress is important, too. I also tell my patients to try to avoid contact with sick people and to avoid subjecting themselves to temperature extremes—as mentioned above, some MS symptoms become very prominent when the patient becomes overheated.

Many patients gravitate toward special diets. Several of my patients told me they read that omega-3 and GLA supplements (fish oils) have been shown to reduce inflammation. The problem is, to get enough of these healing oils, you have to swallow a lot of capsules, and although they are not expensive, compared to many drugs they are not cheap either. I tell my patients to eat fewer animal products, eat more fish, and consider adding flaxseed products to the morning meal. If they want to add certain foods that they believe are helpful, I say, why not? If they believe a raw soybean diet or a raw food diet is helpful, and they indulge without sacrificing other nutrients, they have my blessing.

Finally, I believe a positive attitude is important. Often, a patient will view this disease as incurable and untreatable, but this is absolutely without foundation! People with MS can live long and enjoyable lives. I am all for looking at the glass half full, and I think not only every patient but every treating physician should do the same. A positive attitude can greatly improve anyone's sense of well-being and may even have a beneficial effect on the course of the disease.

Pregnancy

Because MS generally strikes during the childbearing years, there is always much discussion on whether or not it is wise to try to have a baby. Studies have shown that MS has no adverse effects on pregnancy, labor, or delivery. To the contrary, pregnant women with MS have a 70 percent *less* chance of symptoms than women with MS who are not pregnant. This mimics rheumatoid arthritis, which also has remitting symptoms during pregnancy, again establishing a common link in the autoimmune diseases. But within the first three months after delivery, the rate of recurrence of disease jumps to 70 percent greater than the norm. The rate jump may be because of the elevation in hormones in the first three months in women who are

pregnant and the changes in the immune system that a woman undergoes when she carries a baby. As discussed in detail in chapter 2, a fetus's genes are 50 percent foreign and yet the body does not reject it,
which tells us that the immune system adapts to meet the special
needs exhibited during the gestational period.

Because this is a disease of younger people, many of my patients
with MS ask me whether it is advisable to become pregnant. Unfortunately, there is no stock answer, because each case of MS is individual and each varies according to the patient. For this reason, and
because pregnancy is such a personal issue, I always refer them to
their obstetrician/gynecologist.

What has happened to my four MS patients closely illustrates what
happens to so many patients with the disease. Although these women
had different symptoms, I started all four on the same chemical regimens. I treated them first with an immunosuppressive type of cortisone called *solumedrol*. They received it intravenously over several
days in a high dose, to slow the autoimmune process. Then I placed
them on a regimen of subcutaneous interferon beta over several
months. They have not all responded alike, however. Ann has left the
magazine and has just signed a contract to write a book about the
fashion industry. She is doing well and has been symptom-free for
two years now. So has Cynthia, who next week moves to Tuscany
with her chef husband. Jane has had another baby, and afterward her
symptoms escalated. She has trouble with movement, and fatigue
continues to dog her, but she knows how to schedule her day and
seems to be getting along as well as can be expected. She responded
well to another run of steroids and then interferon. Sara is working as
an assistant district attorney. She, too, has days when she feels tired,
but she has never again experienced a memory loss, and, in fact, is
one of those people who always knows where her keys are.

The Future of Multiple Sclerosis

The good thing about MS, if we can look at the bright side, is that unlike most of the autoimmune diseases for which there are many different antigens to defend against, with MS, we know that the antigen
is myelin basic protein. This knowledge allows us to try a new

method of treatment called immune tolerance. The theory is as follows: Giving a patient a small amount of a specific substance over a period of time will allow her immune system to become used to its presence, that is, immune tolerant of that substance. Some of my colleagues have been giving myelin basic protein by mouth to their MS patients for just that purpose. In other words, if myelin is the antigen, and if you give a person enough myelin basic protein, either by vein or mouth, the immune system will become so familiar with it, it will no longer think of it as foreign matter and will eventually ignore it. Unfortunately, like many other treatments under investigation, at this point using immune tolerance to treat MS is better in theory than in practice.

Along the same vein, a group of Boston physicians investigated a similar approach using chicken collagen in patients with rheumatoid arthritis. The collagen was fed by mouth to countless volunteers in an effort to protect them against human collagen, one of the targets of the immune system in rheumatoid arthritis. (Aha! At last, a possible explanation for the magical healing powers of chicken soup!) While this, too, had less-than-hoped-for results, the principle of tolerance induction continues to be tried in many of the autoimmune diseases, from diabetes to lupus.

It is continually intriguing to researchers that MS is found four times as often in women than men. Accordingly, the National Multiple Sclerosis Society has initiated research projects that investigate the effects of hormones on brain growth and function. Recent research on rats that have allergic encephalitis—a nonautoimmune disease that also causes demyelination—indicates that estrogen at certain doses actually improves the disease. This prompted a considerable search for some of the effects of other sex hormones in the control of this disease.

The most interesting aspect of the new therapeutics for MS is, not surprisingly, the control of cytokines. Other new therapies include an oral form of interferon, monoclonal antibodies directed against cytokines, bone marrow transplantation, and T-cell vaccination (a method to block certain antigens from activating the immune system). With all this, I am very hopeful that we will see a cure for this condition in my lifetime. Very hopeful indeed.

CHAPTER SEVEN

PANDAS

The Jekyll and Hyde Syndrome

S OMETIMES I MARVEL at how far the field of medicine has come since I first entered it in 1973. Other times, I can only wish we were further along. One of those times was several years ago when I first met Pam, a rail-thin eleven-year-old girl, and her parents. At our first meeting, Pam appeared to be a typical preadolescent child, blond hair pulled into a ponytail, mouth full of braces, her smile just one degree of shy. The only indication that anything might be wrong with this child was the not-so-subtle motion she exhibited during our interview—every so often her fingers would play an invisible piano in her lap.

Their pediatrician sent the family to me because he suspected Pam had PANDAS, a childhood autoimmune disease. But he said he wanted an immunologist to make the definitive diagnosis and to treat her. When I asked Pam's mother to relate her daughter's recent history, she got right to the point:

"It all happened so suddenly," she told me. "She hadn't been sick at all. In fact, her brother Michael had strep throat two weeks before, and we were just happy Pam didn't get it. Then, out of nowhere, she started to make these strange, sporadic movements. First, it was her leg, then her fingers. Initially, we put them down as muscle spasms. Perhaps she was working too hard at soccer practice, or maybe it was growing pains. But every time I wanted to talk to her about it, she refused and would storm up to her room to avoid the discussion, which is not at all like her. She usually is a very calm and soft-spoken child. But while I attributed *that* behavior to her being preadolescent, I have to admit my husband and I were becoming increasingly perplexed.

"Two days later it was as if the child I sent off to school that morning was not the same one who came home that afternoon," she said. "She came into the house, slammed the door behind her, and announced she wasn't going back to school because the kids were making fun of her. She said that the teacher thought she was faking the movements just to get out of class. She claimed that there were too many germs at school for her to be safe, and she was suddenly afraid to hold someone's paper or even to touch the chalk." Pam's teacher had called late that afternoon to report that Pam had spent much of the day in the bathroom washing her hands and indeed, that evening, she could barely come to the dinner table for all the repeating rituals. At that point, both parents realized something must be done, and quickly.

The early diagnosis of this syndrome was not difficult because there are only a few conditions that can cause choreiform movements (the sudden thrusting or jerking of her legs or piano-playing motions with the fingers) associated with obsessive-compulsive disorder (repetitive behavior, such as handwashing, and persistence of phobias, such as fear of heights and germs). When the patient is a child and the symptoms are preceded by a strep infection, you most assuredly are dealing with PANDAS. The only confounding issue was that Pam had not had strep throat. Or so we thought.

What Is PANDAS?

PANDAS, which is an acronym for pediatric autoimmune neuropsychiatric disorders associated with streptococcal infections, generally affects prepubescent children. The disease is set in motion when the child contracts an infection known as group A beta hemolytic streptococcal infection, otherwise known as strep throat. When this happens, the child's body begins to produce antibodies against the disease, the natural sequence of events. Unfortunately, in a subset of vulnerable children, the immune system goes awry and in addition to attacking the strep bacteria, the antibodies attack structures in their bodies that are similar to the strep bacteria.

As far as we know, only two organs in the body contain specific areas in which the molecular makeup of the tissue closely resembles strep bacteria. These are the valves of the heart and the basal ganglia, two pistachio-nut-size areas deep within the brain, which are responsible for both behavior and movement. When the antibodies cross-react with the heart valves, the consequence is rheumatic fever (see chapter 8), which can generate a heart murmur, tremors, arthritis, and Sydenham's chorea (short, purposeless movements, muscular weakness, and sporadic emotional problems). But when the brain cells of the basal ganglia are the targets, as in PANDAS, the result is a tic-like behavior similar to Tourette's syndrome and usually also bizarre psychiatric behavior, such as obsessive-compulsive disorder (OCD). Even more disquieting is the fact that the symptoms of PANDAS always come on suddenly and dramatically, as Pam's did, perhaps as quickly as overnight.

Clearly, not every child who experiences strep throat will get PANDAS. Because the disease has only recently been defined, and indeed is still in the process of definition, we can only estimate the numbers of children who are stricken with this disease; the current calculations are at less than 1 percent of children who get strep throat. I do not believe we have yet made the scientific connection to many of its psychological manifestations, however, which would probably send this number higher.

The Discovery of PANDAS: A History Lesson

Like so many other scientific discoveries, the discovery of PANDAS as we know it was made in the course of searching for something else. The sequence of events were set in motion by Dr. Ralph Williams, a former Rockefeller University scientist and colleague from Albuquerque, New Mexico, who in the early 1970s first described anti-brain-nucleus antibodies (antibodies that cross-react with the brain) following strep infection and their correlation with chorea in people with acute rheumatic fever (RF). Then, in the late 1980s, Dr. Susan Swedo and her colleague Dr. Judith Rappaport were studying children with acute rheumatic fever who also had Sydenham's chorea. While conducting this research, they observed that many of the children who had chorea also had OCD symptoms.

In a 1994 scientific paper, Drs. Swedo and Rappaport noted that in one retrospective study and two prospective studies, about three-quarters of the children with Sydenham's chorea had acute-onset obsessive-compulsive symptoms. Further, in a group of fifty-four children who were treated for childhood onset OCD, one-third also had the choreiform movements attendant to Sydenham's chorea. When these children came back for followup visits two to seven years later, the behavioral symptoms were gone. This led the researchers to hypothesize that perhaps the same disease, or cause of the disease, was responsible for both the behavioral symptoms and the abnormal neurologic signs.

They immediately started looking at the differences between the manifestations of the OCD in children who, like the others, had had strep, but not necessarily RF. There was a marked difference in the way the OCD presented itself in each group. In a large percentage of the children, the OCD came on suddenly, as opposed to coming on gradually and then waxing and waning, which is the normal course. This group also had an earlier age of onset. These and other manifestations led them to identify this subset of children as having PANDAS. It was actually one of Dr. Swedo's assistants who came up with the name "PANDAS" in an effort to make it easier for the young children to explain their disease to others.

Diagnosing PANDAS

So far, the best way to diagnose PANDAS is clinically, that is, based on observation and/or a litany of a child's symptoms. To date, there are no laboratory tests that can definitively diagnose the disease. We do employ laboratory techniques to positively identify the preexisting strep infection, however. This is done by culturing bacteria taken from the throat during the time of the active infection, or by blood test after the strep symptoms of fever and sore throat have subsided. The blood test allows us to look for an elevated titer (strength of antibody), in this case an antistrep titer, which tells us that the infection existed at some point within the past few months and that the child created antibodies to fight it. Antibodies can stay in the body, sometimes for months after an infection has disappeared. The amount of time they remain behind will vary by individual. (Just to clarify things, I would like to note that antibodies to diseases have a relatively short life in the body. It is the immune system's *memory* of a disease that lasts forever. This means that if a virus, such as chickenpox, should reenter the body a second time, the immune system immediately recognizes it and calls the antibodies for that disease to start reproducing themselves as a means of defense.)

Dr. Swedo and others at the National Institutes of Mental Health (NIMH) have described five clinical symptoms that lead to a diagnosis of PANDAS:

▷ A patient must exhibit clear signs of OCD and/or a tic disorder.

▷ A patient's symptoms must be observed first prior to the onset of puberty.

▷ The symptoms must come on abruptly, which differs considerably from the typical chronic nature of other tic disorders and OCD.

▷ Symptoms must always follow strep infections. In some cases the OCD shows up quite a while past the point when strep titers are detectable. When that happens, it is necessary to wait for the next strep or upper respiratory infection (URI) to see if tics or OCD are exacerbated by the illness, in which case PANDAS is the likely diagnosis. It is equally important to determine that the child is free of symptoms when there is *no* strep infection.

▷ There must be some neurologic abnormalities, such as choreiform movements, as well as remarkable changes in the child's disposition, behavior, or attention span.

Although these five criteria are clear, definitive symptomatic diagnosing of PANDAS can still get tricky. That is because not every child with OCD has PANDAS, although almost every child with PANDAS has some form of OCD. Likewise, every child with PANDAS will have some form of tic or abrupt motion disorder similar to Tourette's syndrome, yet not every child with Tourette's has PANDAS. In children with non-PANDAS-related tics or OCD, the symptoms manifest themselves at a relatively consistent level. An episodic course for a child with PANDAS, however, begins suddenly and dramatically and is followed by a slow, gradual improvement (over weeks or months or even longer) until the symptoms are no longer apparent. In addition, the child will remain symptom-free until he or she until gets another strep infection or URI, after which symptoms will suddenly return. There is no way of knowing for how long PANDAS will continue to befall any patient.

The symptoms that Pam displayed were classic. Her abrupt outbursts, repeated fear of germs, and frequent trips to the bathroom to wash her hands are concordant with the diagnosis of OCD. The pianist-like movements of her fingers and her leg tremors are consistent with chorea. In addition, her behavioral change, which came on suddenly, was inconsistent with that of the calm and friendly child she was described as by her parents.

What made her disease a bit harder to diagnose was the fact that she had never complained of a sore throat and could not remember having had one in the recent past. Yet, a blood evaluation showed that she did indeed have titers for strep, which we assumed she had contracted from her brother, but perhaps in an unusually mild form. Or, perhaps because of her easygoing nature, it was altogether possible that she simply had not complained about the strep when she had it.

To acquire PANDAS, a child must have precisely the right immune response genes on chromosome 6 (see chapter 2). In other words, without the right genetic markers—and mercifully this is rare—the illness will pass her by. To reiterate: Less than 1 percent of children who get a strep infection will get PANDAS. I suppose you could say that's the good news.

Treating PANDAS

There is no true therapy for PANDAS. Currently, two methods are in use, both of which treat the symptoms by attempting to remove faulty antibodies from the blood. The first procedure, *plasmapheresis,* filters the blood plasma in an effort to weed out specific antigen/antibody complexes. The procedure is similar to dialysis, which is used for people with chronic renal failure to cleanse their blood of poisonous waste. With the child in a bed or chair, blood is drawn through a narrow tube and passed into a machine where it is filtered and reinfused into the child. Usually, this is done once to twice a week, and the course of treatment can be completed in a month's time. Then the child is evaluated to determine whether there is significant change in behavior.

The second method involves an intravenous infusion of immunoglobulin (IVIG), which is pooled antibody that is synthesized in a laboratory and is given to treat some autoimmune diseases. No one really understands how IVIG works, but it seems to be very effective at removing, or at least disarming, pathologic antibodies in people who have these syndromes.

These two procedures are currently in controlled clinical trials to gauge their effectiveness and compare one against the other. So far, they both seem to be effective, at least in reducing the severity of the OCD, but I admit that I wish there were better solutions. In any case, left untreated, the symptoms of PANDAS will eventually subside, at least until the immune system is challenged by another strep infection.

Many parents of my patients ask me why the drugs we use against strep are not used to treat PANDAS. Unfortunately, those drugs—primarily antibiotics—are useless against this disease, because the problem is not the strep-related bacteria but rather the antibodies made in response to them. By the time the immune system decides to attack the basal ganglia—generally a week or two after the start of the infection and often longer—the organisms for strep bacteria are long gone. Parents also inquire if there is anything they can do if their child has strep, to prevent the disease from affecting their child. To date, there is nothing I know of that can be done to thwart PANDAS in a child with strep infection, but I believe just being aware of this disease is important so that you can recognize it if it should occur.

A Final Note on PANDAS

To me, PANDAS is among the most challenging of the autoimmune disorders, in large measure because it holds the human mind hostage to its actions. I cannot imagine a clearer or more tragic example of the havoc one simple antibody can cause than to produce a psychosis in a child. Nor, as a parent myself, can I imagine how overwhelmingly frightening it must be to send your little girl off to school and watch a stranger come home. In fact, it is when I see what dreadful trials can beset a child that I know why I chose immunology and not pediatrics as my vocation.

Fortunately, PANDAS remains equally intriguing to scientists. Many continue to study the etiology of the disease in an effort to answer some of the many questions that are associated with it. For example, we know that strep causes PANDAS. But not *all* strep causes PANDAS. What identifies the particular strain of strep that is the culprit? More important, why are some children protected from this disease and not all? Are there other neurochemical factors associated with this illness? Does drug treatment help or does it just mask the symptoms? Does this phenomenon run in families; that is, do the genes that are responsible for the antigenic confusion show up regularly in a particular family?

Because the entire issue of the way brain cells cross-react with antibodies is still so new, no one is completely sure of all its manifestations. Physicians are beginning to suspect that many of the psychological syndromes that show up in childhood, including anorexia and attention deficit disorder, might have autoimmunity as their basis. On a greater scale, the tendency of one disease to play a role in another is also being given a new consideration. For example, I pointed out earlier in this chapter that following rheumatic fever, many but not all patients develop uncontrolled tremors. It turns out that that same type (that is to say, we believe they are of a similar type) of tremors or chorea are found in antiphospholipid (sticky blood) syndrome (see chapter 3). Although this hypothesis continues to be very controversial, I have always believed that the two conditions are connected, thus making antiphospholipid syndrome a strep-related disease.

I also believe that the more we understand about the scientific manifestations of diseases such as PANDAS, the more we'll know about the role of the immune system in neuropsychiatric disorders, and ultimately the deeper we will be able to peer into the brain and understand the way it functions. This view may be limited for now, but any information that emerges will clearly be advantageous, both in the diagnosis as well as in the treatments for these disorders in children and adults. At least I am hoping this will be so.

CHAPTER EIGHT

STREPTOCOCCAL INFECTION AND RHEUMATIC FEVER

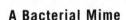

A Bacterial Mime

HE OLD WOMAN used to walk quickly and purposefully across the campus of Rockefeller University. She was short and heavyset with snow-white hair, much like my grandmother, but unlike my grandmother, she had a huge impact on science, medicine, and the history of the world. On the way to lunch daily, we crossed paths. I recognized her, but I also knew from living in New York City that it is not politically correct to stare at those who are famous, so I always kept on going. She was, after all, the great Rebecca Lancefield, responsible for a good part of modern-day strep microbiology.

Dr. Lancefield is credited with discovering the key to identifying streptococcus bacteria and classifying the more than sixty strains of streptococci in a system that is still in use today. She proved, as well, that the same strep bacteria *group A* could cause a number of conditions, from sore throats to scarlet fever, a discovery that ultimately would have a mammoth impact on the field of rheumatology. Doctor Lancefield began teaching microbiology at Rockefeller in 1922 and remained there as an active scientist until her death in 1981 at the age of eighty-six. To this day I stand in awe of this woman who spent her life making organisms her friends and placing them in the context of disease, and, subsequently, history.

The importance of group A streptococcal infection cannot be overstated. It remains one of the largest killers in the world. The strep bug produces a toxin that can ravage the body overnight with fever, sore throat, and excruciating pain. When left untreated, it can beget a cat-and-mouse game with the immune system that wreaks irreversible havoc on one or more of the body's organs. We saw this happen to an unsuspecting little girl in chapter 7 on PANDAS. In that occurrence, the strep so closely mimicked the tissue of the basal ganglia (in the brain) that when the immune system geared up to go after the strep, it also, mistakenly, went after the tissue in the brain, attacking it as though it were the strep bug itself, and leaving the child with psychiatric and movement problems. Untreated strep can also result in a disease called *rheumatic fever* that affects the heart.

What Is Rheumatic Fever?

Rheumatic fever (RF) is an inflammatory disease that can develop after an infection with streptococcus bacteria (such as strep throat or scarlet fever). Unlike PANDAS, which affects only the brain, rheumatic fever manifests itself in many areas of the body, including the heart, joints, skin, and brain. In other words, when the immune system thinks it is attacking the strep, it is actually invading these other self-tissues. The symptoms most common to rheumatic fever are as follows:

▷ *Arthritis of the large joints.* Rheumatic-fever-related arthritis is generally the earliest symptom of this disease. It can affect several joints in progression or can be *polyarticular* and affect many joints simultaneously. The inflammation and pain from arthritis can be acute, but these symptoms go away when treated with anti-inflammatory drugs and analgesics.

▷ *Chorea.* Sydenham's chorea, or "St. Vitus' dance," is a neurologic manifestation of this disease. Patients periodically exhibit rapid and involuntary movements, muscle weakness, and sometimes emotional disturbances.

▷ *Erythema marginatum.* This rheumatic-fever-induced rash, which is always temporary, produces redness and scaling that extends across the trunk of the body, arms, and legs.

▷ *Subcutaneous nodules.* These small, hard, painless areas are comprised of fibrous tissue. They arise under the skin, generally over the bony structures, and generally dissolve when the disease is treated.

▷ *Rheumatic heart disease.* This is the most dangerous of the symptoms of rheumatic fever. It occurs when the strep antigen cross-reacts with heart tissue, producing *carditis*—an inflammation of the heart muscle—and valvular damage, which can lead to congestive heart failure and pericarditis (inflammation of the outer lining of the heart). The most perilous aspect of rheumatic fever is its ability to scar the heart's valves (most commonly the mitral valve, which lies between the two left chambers of the heart), which occurs in more than 50 percent of cases. This scarring can stiffen the valve—a condition called *stenosis*—and make it more difficult for the valve to open properly or to close completely. In turn, the heart has to work harder each time it pumps blood to the rest of the body. Mitral valve stenosis can lead to backed-up blood in the heart and ultimately to congestive heart failure, an acutely dangerous clinical syndrome that must be treated quickly and aggressively with a combination of diuretics and anti-inflammatory drugs, or with valve replacement surgery.

It is important to note that rheumatic fever does not occur every time a strep infection goes untreated. It happens in fewer than 3 percent of people who have rheumatic fever. The average duration of an attack of acute rheumatic fever is three months or longer. After the acute attack has subsided, many people are left with damaged heart valves (*rheumatic heart disease*), and some will have recurrent attacks of acute rheumatic fever, frequently causing even greater damage to the heart valves. Today, this disease is far more common worldwide than in the United States. It primarily affects children between the ages of six and fifteen and generally occurs within one to five weeks following infection with strep. In up to one-third of cases, the streptococcal infection is symptom-free, so that many people do not even know they have the disease.

Hoda's Story

An acute case of rheumatic fever is what brought Hoda, a seventeen-year-old Egyptian girl, and her aunt to my office four years ago. Hoda is from Cairo, a place where time stands still for many poor peasants, and diseases that were eradicated from the West many years ago still ravage families. While rheumatic fever affects people from all over the world, the disease has a particularly strong foothold in countries such as Iraq and Egypt, where strep illnesses are all but epidemic. Hoda's doctor, whom I had met on an earlier visit to Egypt, sent her to the United States to see me; he knew her uncle was wealthy enough to fly her here for an evaluation by a rheumatologist. In her records, which arrived the week before she did, Hoda's doctor outlined the panoply of her symptoms: severe arthritis, a bizarre rash, high fever, occasional involuntary movements of her arms, and what he called a "highly abnormal EKG." Typical of the way rheumatic fever operates, Hoda's symptoms had broken out three weeks after her strep throat subsided.

When I first saw her in my office, she appeared a very quiet, frail-looking, gangly young woman. She wore a white shirt, khakis, and sneakers that reminded me of a GAP advertisement. Her aunt was more formally dressed and was far more adept than Hoda at conversation. From the aunt's explanation, it seemed that Hoda was experiencing many of the distressing components of rheumatic fever. She described jerky arm movements and leg movements on only one side of her body. (The location of the movements depends on which side of the brain is involved.) She also told me that Hoda was having problems with the other children in school, who thought her uncontrolled movements were freakish. In the Middle Ages these types of disjointed movements—and those associated with epilepsy—were thought to be a sign of possession by the devil. I could only imagine what that must have been like for this lovely child sitting across from me.

Hoda's symptoms were wholly conspicuous. She had an *erythema marginatum* rash, red, with a deep vermilion border, in full bloom on her face and arms. Her eyelids looked heavy, and it was clear she was struggling to keep them open. Every so often her elbow would fly up from her side like a chicken flapping a wing, or her arm would lift and her fingers dance in the air. How she managed to travel so many hours from Egypt, feeling so ill, was beyond my comprehension, especially since she still had a fever, but her aunt explained that she had slept during much of the journey.

Diagnosing Hoda's Disease

Because there are so many different manifestations of rheumatic fever, there is no specific test that can definitively establish a diagnosis. In my examining room, I did a careful physical examination, first listening to her heart. The rubbing sound I heard led me to suspect that Hoda's heart was enlarged. She also had a diastolic murmur, a sound that showed that her valve was leaking when the ventricle relaxed to accept fresh blood from the lungs. Her rosy cheeks, so common in mitral stenosis, were another major clue to her illness. Of course, many people have rosy cheeks and do not have rheumatic fever; however, the presence of rosy cheeks and a loud mitral opening snap is virtually diagnostic of this disease.

Her rash was clearly related to her disease, and this, along with the choreiform movements, left no doubt that the diagnosis was rheumatic fever. I did a blood workup. The *antistreptolysin test* for toxins and other tests for infectious microbes confirmed my suspicions, and the rest was relatively easy. It is interesting that in the eighteenth century, physicians used only symptoms and signs to make this diagnosis without modern immunology or our twenty-first-century equipment. I admire what must have been their extraordinary clinical talent.

Treating Hoda

Because Hoda looked so frail and ill, I immediately put her into the hospital on bed rest. I prescribed aspirin as well as an anti-inflammatory drug for her joint pains, and loaded her up with intravenous antibiotics.

These would eradicate any group A streptococcus bacteria that remained in her body and prevent the spread of the organism to anyone who was in close contact with her. The antibiotics would forestall a resurgence of strep activity but would do nothing for the immune response that was already in progress.

Hoda began improving immediately. In less than a week, her rash faded, her choreiform movements disappeared, and her arthritis went away, so I took her off the antibiotics. I kept her on aspirin to prevent further inflammation, particularly because at this point I realized it was the inflammation that was causing all the problems. Unfortunately, she continued to experience first-degree heart block (a series of pauses in the electrical conduction system of the heart) from the infection, and the mitral stenosis remained, so that blood flow through the left side of her heart continued to be significantly diminished. I knew just from listening with my stethoscope that her heart murmur was severe.

To get a definitive picture of what was going on inside Hoda's heart, the cardiologist performed a catheterization. This process is also called *cine angiogram* or *angiography*. He first inserted a catheter into an artery in her groin and then slid it up into her left ventricle. Next, he injected a dye and followed its progress in Hoda's heart on X-ray. He could see the function of her heart valves as the dye passed through them. He also did an echocardiogram, which always reminds me of looking for submarines under the sea, since the technology is somewhat the same. An echocardiogram is a test of the sounds of the heart that, when translated on paper, appear as dancing shadows.

Both tests confirmed just what we suspected: Hoda had a very stiff, tight valve that did not open sufficiently to let the required amount of blood through. The blood was being pumped into her heart at a less-than-normal rate, and because it could not get through the valve easily, it could not be pumped out of her heart fast enough. As a result, some of the blood began to back up into her lungs. It was a classic, textbook case of mitral valve stenosis.

It was clear at that point that the only way to restore her heart to normal was to replace the damaged valve. The only question was when. Heart surgery is a major procedure for anyone, but in one so ill as Hoda, it is doubly so. A cardiologist and a cardiac surgeon saw her, and they decided it was best to schedule her for open-heart surgery before she returned to Egypt. For several days, while she waited for her surgery, I could hardly keep the medical students from holding court in her room. They all wanted to hear the heart and the chest sounds that resulted from this disease, which has almost been eradicated in the West.

Ten days after she entered the hospital, Hoda underwent a valve replacement. The surgeon put in a pig valve that hopefully will serve her for many years to come. This is a far cry from the way valve surgery was performed when I was an intern. Then, the chest would barely be opened, the heart cut into and the stiff valve leaflets would be "cracked" like an egg—sometimes with the introduction of a finger—to expand the opening and allow blood to flow through.

Hoda remained in the hospital for another week, and then we made plans for her to be discharged. I advised her to take penicillin daily for five years as a prophylactic against a recurrence. People who have suffered a case of rheumatic fever have a tendency to develop flareups, with repeated streptococcal infections. Recurrence is relatively common in the absence of maintenance on low-dose antibiotics, particularly during the first three to five years after the first rheumatic-fever episode. I faxed a summary of her case to her doctor in Cairo and called him to make sure he was current on her situation, because I find that teenagers tend not to be very compliant about these kinds of things, and it would take careful monitoring to ensure that Hoda followed my wishes. This was essential for her, because going back to her country—the very place where the infection began—put her at risk.

Some Additional Thoughts

The similarity between rheumatic fever and other autoimmune illnesses is startling. The symptoms are often compared to those of diseases such as antiphospholipid syndrome or multiple sclerosis. Strep has been invoked for years as a potential cause of these conditions. We simply cannot get a handle on what it is that makes these other diseases so similar to rheumatic fever. Many scientists believe that all of autoimmunity is about mimicry, that the chameleon-like nature of bacteria and viruses is well known, and that all autoimmune diseases are related to mechanisms such as this one. The true difference is that, thanks to the dedication of Dr. Rebecca Lancefield, we know about the strep bug, and we can both isolate it and prove its presence. We cannot yet do that with the villains in many of these other devastating diseases. In fact, we do not even know what most of them are.

CHAPTER NINE

VASCULITIS

Destroyed Pipes

NURSES ARE NOT supposed to get sick. But Terry, a twenty-nine-year-old charge nurse for the intensive care unit (ICU) at a New York City hospital, unwittingly became an exception to the rule. On the morning she became ill, Terry bounded out of bed with great expectations. This was, after all, her first weekend off in a month, and she had very much been looking forward to it. Eager to get out into the morning sunshine, she pulled on her shorts and shirt, laced her new running shoes, gulped down a bottle of water, and headed out into the glorious October day. Jogging toward Central Park, she waved to some friends as they passed. She ran into the park through the Seventy-ninth Street entrance at 8:25 A.M. on her watch and started south. About ten minutes into her run, aware of nothing but the leaves falling around her, she suddenly felt a wave of nausea. It was a subtle discomfort, lasting a brief moment. Continuing on, she considered what she might have eaten the day before that might have caused it, but could not think of anything in particular. Twenty minutes later, as Terry turned right just north of the

Wollman Skating Rink, she experienced another wave of nausea, only this time it was accompanied by a sharp pain in her head. This time, she thought of her patients in the ICU, many of whom had major infections, and wondered if she might have caught a bug from one of them. But she knew doctors and nurses quite often believe that they have caught some illness or other from their patients, and she decided not to fall into that trap. In another five minutes, Terry's eyes began to bother her. She slowed her pace, pulled off her sunglasses, and rubbed them with her shirt to clear the sudden blur, but in fact it was her eyes, not the glasses, that were at fault.

As the pain in her head accelerated, Terry did something very rare for her—she stopped running.

Walking back uptown, Terry vomited twice. She barely made it to the door of her apartment, where, sweating profusely, she passed out. A neighbor discovered her on the floor and called 911. The emergency medical technicians (EMTs) found her babbling incoherently and hot to the touch. They started an intravenous line, stabilized her vital signs as best they could, then rushed her to the nearest hospital, which just happened to be the one in which she worked.

By the time she arrived at the ER, Terry was ashen, still incoherent, and had spiked a temperature of 105 degrees. She could not move her left leg and had trouble lifting her right hand. The triage nurse, seeing these seizure-like symptoms, immediately admitted her as a level one (the highest) emergency. The priority with a first-time seizure is to find the cause, which can include a blow to the head, a brain tumor, a vascular malformation, a stroke, or a metabolic reaction to drugs, both legal and illegal. The ER staff sprang into action. The first priority was to bring down Terry's spiking fever, which they did, if only temporarily, with Tylenol and a cooling blanket. Next, they administered drugs to lower her blood pressure, which was on the rise and, if left unchecked, could precipitate a stroke. All this took almost an hour. While the ER nurses tried to stabilize Terry's vital signs, the ER doctors conferred about whether or not to start antibiotic therapy immediately. They were worried that she might have meningitis, in which case every second counted. Still, they knew the importance of first taking cultures of her blood, urine, spinal fluid, and sputum for evaluation, because once antibiotics have been started, there is no hope of getting a true reading about any disease from a culture.

Within an hour, her vital signs were stable and her breathing under control, but Terry continued to show signs of incoherence and sporadic jerkiness in her leg. The ER doctor called in specialists from the infectious disease (ID) and neurology departments. The neurology resident arrived first and quickly arranged for a CAT scan. This would tell her if Terry had bled into her brain or had a massive bacterial infection. Bacteria in the brain tissue or spinal fluid can cause pus to form, and when a patient has profound neurological signs and is running a high fever, as Terry was, this is a good possibility. If that were the case, the official diagnosis would be meningitis, which could also account for Terry's high fever, seizure, and headache. But the CAT scan turned out to be normal. The next place to look for signs of infection was in the spinal fluid. Because time was of the essence, the neurologist performed a lumbar puncture and took the spinal fluid to the laboratory for evaluation herself. All anyone could do now was wait for the results of the tests. In the meantime, Terry was transferred from the ER to the ICU, where she would be closely observed and continuously evaluated.

As Terry was wheeled into the ICU, five staff members, advised earlier that "one of their own" was on the way, stood at the doorway to the unit, waiting to help in any way they could. In any hospital unit, where working conditions are so close, a seriously ill colleague affects everyone. Terry was quickly transferred to a hospital bed where, amid a flurry of activity, IV lines were added, and several wires connected machines to her body in order to monitor her heart rate and blood pressure. For the rest of the day she lay still, the only sound in her room the beeping of the monitors and the low din of voices of the physicians and nurses who attended her.

Results from the laboratory tests came back the next day. They showed that Terry did not have enough cells in her spinal fluid to make the case for meningitis, and no bacterial infections were present in her blood or spinal fluid. In fact, not a single test came back positive. The whole picture just did not make sense. For five more days, Terry's fever vacillated between 101°F and 105°F. Both the neurologists and the infectious disease specialists were stymied. Terry was still incoherent at times, and there was no obvious evidence of the origin of her infection. As her condition continued to deteriorate, the cardiologists were summoned to evaluate a recently developed heart murmur, and the hematologists were called because her blood counts dropped precipitously.

That first week, Terry remained in a state of periodic sleep and wakefulness. The medical staff remained frustrated and bewildered by her situation and could not do much more than run tests and watch as the IVs dripped medications and nourishment into their patient's body.

Then, on the eighth day of her hospitalization, a good friend, an ICU nurse from another hospital, paid her a visit. As she sat with Terry and held her hand, she noticed very faint, multiple splinter-like hemorrhages under Terry's fingernails. The friend called in another nurse and within the hour, they both watched, dumbfounded, as Terry began to break out in small, dark gangrenous spots at the tips of her ears, fingers, and toes. The infectious disease specialist returned and examined her again, and, he said later, "a light over my head went on." It occurred to him that these particular symptoms, while often seen in blood infections, could also be evidence of a not-so-rare but very elusive autoimmune disease. "If I were a betting man," he told the nurses, "I'd put my money on vasculitis."

What Is Vasculitis?

The term *vasculitis* means inflammation of the blood vessels. In autoimmune vasculitis, antibodies attack segments of the inner walls of the blood vessels—the *endothelium*—provoking a situation that can seriously affect the flow of blood. During the attack, the antibodies chew away the *elastin*, a substance within the vessel wall that normally keeps the vessel tight and smooth. With the elastin gone, the vessel wall becomes weak and balloons out, leaving in its path a microaneurysm (an out-pouching in the wall of the vessel), or more likely, a series of microaneurysms that vary in size and often are no larger than the letter "O."

Every vessel in the cardiovascular system—veins, arteries, and capillaries—is fair game for these antibodies, which means that every vessel in the body is open to attack. Vasculitis can disrupt any organ system, including the central and peripheral nervous systems, which is where it first affected Terry. The condition can be localized to a single organ, or it can be systemic and involve many organs. No matter, the result is a panoply of symptoms, depending on which blood vessels are involved and which organs are affected.

Terry was initially diagnosed with vasculitis of the central nervous system that manifested itself first as a cerebral vasculitis (vasculitis of the brain). Because it was not associated with any other diseases, it was considered primary vasculitis. Vasculitis can occur alongside both autoimmune and non-autoimmune diseases, in which case it is called secondary vasculitis. Some non-autoimmune diseases that are associated with vasculitis include coronary artery disease and hepatitis, but I have seen vasculitis caused by drug allergies, infections, and strep throat. I have also seen it occur for no obvious reason at all.

Terry's disease began as inflammation in several areas of her circulatory system, including the vessels of her brain, which is what caused her incoherence. The splinter hemorrhages beneath her nails were the results of microinfarctions, that is, clogging of small blood vessels in those peripheral areas. The purple or gangrenous patches on her fingers and the tips of her ears are called vasculitic lesions. These resulted from a lack of oxygen to the tissues, causing a slow necrosis (death) of the compromised tissue.

The many forms of primary vasculitis include the following:

> ▷ *Giant cell arteritis.* This rare condition affects people over fifty and typically involves the medium to large blood vessels that supply the head and neck.
> ▷ *Temporal arteritis.* A common type of vasculitis that affects older people; 25 percent of people with giant cell arteritis also have temporal arteritis.
> ▷ *Polyarteritis nodosa.* The prototype of systemic vasculitis, this involves many different organ systems and focused on medium-size arteries.
> ▷ *Takayasu's arteritis.* A large-vessel vasculitis, this sometimes affects the internal organs and usually occurs in women younger than fifty.
> ▷ *Wegener's granulomatosis.* A systemic disease, this type encompasses the lungs, kidneys, upper respiratory tract, and other organs, but rarely the blood vessels to the brain.

▷ *Buerger's disease.* This disease affects the blood flow to the fingers and toes, and, when compromised, can lead to gangrene.

▷ *Kawasaki's disease.* A very rare form of vasculitis, Kawaski's occurs in children from two months up to twelve years of age, but can occur in adults. Symptoms begin with lethargy and progress to fever, rash over the trunk, and flulike symptoms. The most perilous aspect of this disease is when the coronary arteries become vasculitic and form aneurysms that can burst and cause death. If diagnosed in time, however, Kawasaki's disease is easily managed with drugs such as aspirin and eventually rescinds (sometimes within a year). Prognosis for complete recovery is excellent.

I for one believe that many of the sudden deaths that we see in young people, such as the early brain hemorrhage of a twenty-five-year-old on drugs or a heart attack on the ice of a thirty-year-old hockey player, might have vasculitis as some part of the cause. Most of these young adults are thought to have genetic weaknesses of the heart muscles and a condition called *cardiomyopathy,* but a fair number of them have the blood-vessel inflammation that follows an infection or other insult to the immune system. Unfortunately, only the pathologist knows for sure.

Diagnosing Vasculitis

Vasculitis is one of the more difficult diagnoses to make. I call it a "wastebasket" diagnosis simply because, as we saw earlier, no one seems to consider it early in the disease-seeking process. So many theories are offered and discarded first, that sometimes just that exercise in itself is enough to tell me what lies ahead. All too often it takes a scientific bent and a Sherlock Holmesian mind to diagnose this disease early in the patient's course.

What tipped off the resident who diagnosed Terry was the fast onset of gangrenous spots on her ears and the splinter hemorrhages under her nails where her capillaries had shut down, stopping the blood flow. It would have been helpful if someone had thought to do an antinuclear antibody (ANA) test, because that would have at least helped determine if this disease was autoimmune-related. But the ER physicians never considered autoimmune disease because Terry's symptoms—fever, nausea, and high blood pressure—almost perfectly mimicked meningitis, hepatitis, and even endocarditis (infection of the inner walls of the heart). So everyone thought she had an infection of some sort. In hindsight, of course, it all makes perfect sense. Vasculitis is an acute-onset disease with symptoms that arise suddenly and seemingly from nowhere.

As soon as it became clear her disease might be autoimmune-related, I was called in on Terry's case. Before examining her, I read her hospital chart and evaluated the results of the tests that had already been run. The most revealing was the *magnetic resonance angiogram* (MRA), a test that evaluates the flow of blood within the brain. The results showed blood vessels that, in certain areas, resembled a pearl necklace with inch-long areas that pouched out, crimped, and pouched out again.

Armed with Terry's X-rays and her chart, I went to her hospital room to meet her and examine her. She was lying in the bed with her arms at her side; her eyes were open, staring at the ceiling. As I spoke to her, she shifted her gaze, but I still had to tell her who I was several times before she finally understood. With some patience and effort, I eventually was able to elicit the important information I needed from her medical history. It helped that she was a nurse and familiar with essential medical details. Also in her favor was the fact that until this incident, Terry had been in perfect health.

On examining her, I listened first to her vital signs. Then, scanning her body with my eyes, I noted a series of raised purple spots—purpura—which told me all was not well with her blood supply, not surprising in someone with vasculitis. I wrote an order to have the purpura biopsied, and that was about all I could do at the time. The next day the tissue diagnosis report came back as suggestive of vasculitis, but I wanted to do other tests to confirm it. Late that evening, I returned to the hospital to check on her only to find that Terry's platelets had dropped from 150,000, the normal range, to less than 40,000. While this low number of platelets was not enough to make her bleed, it told me she was terribly *thrombocytopenic* (low platelets) and that something untoward was going on inside. It was not clear if an antibody or an endless array of small blood clots was attacking the platelets. I knew only that changes taking place in Terry's blood-stream were nothing we could ignore, not for a minute.

That same night, as Terry's fever continued to rise, I worked along-side the team of doctors and nurses caring for her. We were all rush-ing to learn as fast as possible what we were dealing with because her frighteningly high fever presented an urgent dilemma. If she had an autoimmune form of vasculitis, then she should be immunosup-pressed immediately with strong drugs such as prednisone, methyl-prednisolone, or cytoxan. But if she had some form of virulent infection, then blocking the functions of her immune system at this time would probably seal her fate.

Luckily, all signs pointed in the same direction: the MRA, the biopsy of her purpura, and the other tests all suggested cerebral ar-teritis. But because this is such a complex disease, I wanted even more confirmation, and so I ordered two more tests. The first was a test that seeks the *antineutrophilic cytoplasmic antibody* (ANCA), and is generally diagnostic of vasculitis, but not specific enough to be defin-itive. The ANCA is a very curious antibody that reacts with one of two specific chemicals within the white cell and produces a specific pattern. I do not often use it because it's very expensive and most hos-pitals do not do it on site.

I also ordered a cryoglobulin test, which indicates that a patient has a high amount of immune complex. The cryoglobulin test can be di-agnostic for vasculitis, providing the patient is positive for hepatitis C, which it turned out that Terry was. In such cases, the immune sys-tem produces antibodies that react at a certain temperature. In other words, we are essentially searching for antibodies that are in the pro-cess of forming immune complexes, which show themselves at a tem-perature lower than that of the body.

In this test, a blood sample is taken and the serum is separated into two tubes. One tube is kept in the cold—on a window ledge (in win-ter) or in a refrigerator—and the other one is kept warm, either in the lab incubator or, as I prefer, under my arm for about thirty minutes. After that time, if the dramatic appearance of a small amount of white fluff becomes apparent in the cold tube, whereas the tube sera in the other remains clear, we know that we have a positive cryoglob-ulin result.

It turned out that Terry did indeed have cryoglobulin in her blood, so we knew that she was making lots of immune complexes and, in fact, we watched them emerge out of the cold serum. Immune complexes elicit inflammatory chemicals and cytokines and ultimately lead to inflammation. The positive cryoglobulin test clinched the diagnosis for us—and allowed us to formulate a treatment plan. Not a minute too soon.

Treating Terry's Disease

Terry's cerebral vasculitis was classified as a medical emergency. In such cases, conventional wisdom is to treat the patient right away with intravenous corticosteroid therapy to slow the attack of the antibodies. We knew that the longer we waited, the greater the chances this young woman would suffer a seizure or a stroke—both of which could disable her permanently.

I immediately put Terry on large doses of intravenous steroids, and decided to keep her on them for three days. While large doses of steroids—I call them industrial-strength doses—stop the immune system cold, they do not necessarily stop the disease from progressing. Even with this therapy, for the next two days Terry continued on the brink of catastrophe. Things were deteriorating fast. Her blood pressure was rising, her temperature was climbing, and her pulse was dangerously fast. The team of doctors and nurses in the ICU worked around the clock trying to keep her vital signs normal. We continued to tend to her runaway fever and put her on strong antibiotics to protect her from some common or obscure infection while her immune system was this severely compromised.

Then, on the third day, as if awakening from a long coma, Terry began to come around. On day four, she became much more alert and her temperature dropped. Three days later, her purpura began to fade, and her ulcers began to heal. I discontinued her antibiotics on day eight, as Terry continued to improve. Her speech gradually returned to normal, and her team of doctors and support staff agreed that she was well enough to go home.

On her last day in the hospital, I went in to say good-bye and found her dressed and sitting on the side of her bed. She smiled broadly and put out her hand to shake mine. She showed no signs of someone who had been so close to the brink, and I decided not to discuss it with her at that time—nor might I ever, unless she asks me. I discharged her on small doses of oral cyclophosphamide, a form of chemotherapy, to keep her immune system in check.

After four weeks, Terry returned to work, although she was still experiencing some side effects of the cyclophosphamide. This included some hair loss and the cessation of her periods, which could mean the possible loss of ovarian function. Terry knows she will always be at risk of developing a malignancy because cyclophosphamide changes the character of one's DNA—which is how chemotherapy works—but she also knows that with this treatment, though it may sometimes be fairly difficult, she has little chance of experiencing again the dangerous situation she was in.

I continue to see Terry in my office. I monitor her blood tests while she remains on chemotherapy and give her liver tests to ensure that her hepatitis C does not flare. In the event that she is eventually free of all symptoms of vasculitis, I will try to treat the hepatitis C with interferon, another antiviral cytokine with which we have had much success, although hepatitis C is not curable.

Most forms of vasculitis can be treated and considerable organ damage avoided if the disease is detected early enough. In fact, almost all diagnosed vasculitic conditions are treatable and result in the complete cure of the patient. Whether or not vasculitis will return after remission depends in large part on the type of vasculitis that is present. For example, some types of vasculitis—such as Henoch-Schönlein purpura (HSP) or small vessel vasculitis caused by antibiotics or antidepressants—tend to be self-limited and resolve on their own. Other forms behave less predictably, returning in about half of the cases. Wegener's granulomatosis, giant cell arteritis, Takayasu's arteritis, microscopic polyangiitis, and other types of vasculitis can flare following remission.

Sometimes flares occur when patients discontinue their medications. Other times they occur when treatments are tapered down in an attempt to avoid side effects. A flare will generally start with symptoms similar to the ones that occurred with the original disease. For example, if a headache was the first symptom at the beginning of giant cell arteritis, then a similar type of headache might herald a recurrence of the disease. If purpura lesions occurred on the legs the first time, then reappearance would probably mean the disease is back. It is important to know what to watch for, because medical treatment can and should be started before serious complications set in.

Inflammation of the blood vessels may be more common than any of us imagine. It is possible that atherosclerosis (the basis for heart attacks, the most common cause of death in our society) begins as a form of vasculitis. If that is true, this manifestation of autoimmunity may actually be quite common, if not as exaggerated as we saw with Terry. Cases of vasculitis are not always as clear-cut as Terry's, and each case manifests in a different way. The way the disease presents itself is complicated, and sometimes, unfortunately, with the rarer forms, such as large-vessel vasculitis, diagnosis is often made at autopsy.

Turkey Research

I had my first exposure to vasculitis when I was a kid in high school. I was about fifteen years old, and as a summer job I cared for a group of research turkeys at a large local drug company. The turkeys would be infected with an organism called *Mycoplasma gallisepticum* that caused brain vasculitis; it affects only turkeys, and is not transmissible to people. I recall coming into the lab the day after we infected the turkeys to find a bunch of nonclucking turkeys with drooping wings. This incident had a lasting impression on me (as you can see) and has, even after all these years, reinforced my belief that infection is at the root of most forms of vasculitis, just as it is for hepatitis C and many other diseases. I think about vasculitis each Thanksgiving Day, but I don't share my thoughts with my family—it clearly would spoil their appetites.

CHAPTER TEN

SYSTEMIC LUPUS ERYTHEMATOSUS

The Red Wolf

NO MATTER HOW long I have been in this business, it still distresses me every time I see a woman, or man for that matter, who has symptoms of autoimmune disease but has languished, undiagnosed, for months and even years. Who is at fault here? Is it the patient, who cannot understand that a slight ache in two knees that earlier bent to bathe a baby might portend a major disease? How could she know? She is a lawyer. Is it the medical profession, for not having enough trained rheumatologists who might—I say *might*—recognize such diseases in a nanosecond? I do not think that, either. Perhaps we physicians simply have too much on our plates. Perhaps there is too much medicine today for all of us to know it all. Indeed, that is why we specialize. One of us learns a lot about a little, the other a little about a lot. We try. We study, we conference, we make rounds. Still, we do not know enough. I forgive myself for this. I hope you will too. And I hope Jessica, whose story follows, understands why it took so long for us to know precisely what she has.

Jessica has lupus. Her first symptoms occurred subtly in the early morning hours, as she sat rocking in a small nursery with stars painted on a pale blue ceiling. There, while the crickets sounded out-side, Jess nursed her newborn infant, Hannah. It was just a slight dull ache in her knees, that first sign. Nothing of concern, of course; just enough to make her shift position, gently, so as not to disturb the baby at her breast. (Is nothing ever really *nothing?*)

Jessica and her husband, James, live an idyllic life in a small town in upstate New York. Both are graduates of Harvard Law School. Both were caught up in the New York City rat race. He was in corpo-rate law, she with a law firm on Wall Street. Then, on September 11, it seemed their world, along with the World Trade Center, came crashing down. For several frantic hours, they were unable to locate their three-year-old son, Jamie, or each other. The boy, and his entire class at nursery school, had been taken to New Jersey when the debris from the Towers fell dangerously close to his school. When she finally got word of his whereabouts, Jess went to pick him up while James went home to wait for his family to return. Still stunned, the normally talkative couple ate dinner in silence and later that night, with Jamie in bed asleep, they made a decision: no more city life.

Three months later James bought and began running a country store, while Jess, now pregnant, relished her job as a stay-at-home mom, devoting time to her small son and volunteering at the local li-brary. With the birth of Hannah, it seemed to Jess that her life was complete. Indeed, it was, until that early morning when, as she rocked her nursing infant, she noticed the pain in her knees.

It was not so strange to feel a pain, but that both knees hurt at the same time made her think that perhaps she had knelt too long on the hard tile while bathing her little boy. The next night, however, Jess's knees hurt again, only now her shoulders hurt, too, and her elbows. Even her neck ached. Certain she was coming down with the flu, she called her parents to come and help with the house and children. No sooner did they arrive than she fell into bed. She stayed there the next day and the next, so weak that it was all but impossible for her even to nurse Hannah.

As each day passed, the pains—not debilitating, just there—would shift from one area of her body to another. She took naps, got up, and even felt better, but soon she found herself longing again for her bed. Occasionally, her eye would feel strange. Her family doctor agreed that it was probably the flu, but because she was nursing, she did not want to take any antibiotics, and together the doctor and patient decided it was best just to wait things out.

The second week, things only got worse; Jess began running a fever of 102°F. At the end of the second week of intermittent fever spikes and unaccountable—if still not debilitating—symptoms, Jess paid a visit to the obstetrician who had delivered Hannah. He examined her and ran some general tests, but they revealed little. His clearly well-meaning nurse suggested to Jess that perhaps she had lost too much blood after the delivery and that some good red meat or iron tablets would bring back her energy. Putting aside her vegetarian leanings, no easy concession, Jess heeded the nurse's advice and she actually ate liver and hamburger on alternating days for a week. Miraculously, it seemed, the pain in her joints subsided. But she was still tired (all new mothers are) and beginning to lose weight over and above the normal postpartum loss (no time to eat a decent meal). In fact, in time she actually started feeling better. Despite a few symptoms here and there, on again–off again, Jess decided that she felt well enough to send her parents home and get on with her life.

Then, on Hannah's four-month birthday, still tired but mercifully pain-free, Jess woke up to find a sizeable rash on her face, hands, and lower legs. At first, it was a deep red color, but by late day, some of the patches began to scale. Stunned by what she saw in the mirror, she called her family doctor, who suggested she see a dermatologist. Because her town was so small, he gave her the name of "a top rash specialist" two hours away in New York City, a dermatologist so "top" that he could fit her in only two weeks later.

When Jess and James saw the doctor, or I should say when the doctor saw Jess, he told her on the spot that he could not be certain, but he thought her rash might be the result of a connective tissue disease. The dermatologist explained that he would need some lab confirmation, but that he was fairly confident he was correct, based on her symptoms, her rash, and because the disease followed so soon after her baby was born. As he is a friend of mine, he called me and asked if I could see Jess and her husband that day to save them a trip back to New York City. I was happy to do so, and arranged for them to come to the office late that afternoon at the end of my regular hours.

When the couple arrived, it did not take me long to determine that the dermatologist had probably been correct in his preliminary diagnosis. Both her history and the physical examination that followed suggested that Jess had lupus. Her joints and skin were not the only affected areas; it appeared that her kidneys were becoming involved as well. Her swollen body was my clue, and my suspicions were confirmed by the urine sample she provided. Kidney involvement, a common lupus symptom, is not immediately life-threatening, but can become so in short order, which always gives cause for concern.

Jess and I returned from the examining room to my office, and James joined us there. After we were seated, I told Jess that I would be doing a few more tests, but I was almost certain she had a disease called lupus and that her symptoms indicated that she had what we refer to as a lupus "flare." When I said that, her face almost took on a brightened look. "I don't know much about that, Dr. Lahita, but I'm just so relieved to know that my symptoms finally have a name."

James, clearly the practical one and also clearly relieved, jumped right in. "Okay, Doctor Lahita," he said. "So what do we do to fix her?"

Ah, were it only as easy as that.

What Is Lupus?

Lupus is a multisystem, multiorgan autoimmune disease that is characterized by the production of antibodies to the components of a cell—including the nucleus, which houses the DNA and the cytoplasm—and other tissues. When you consider that all we are made of is cells, cells held together by a fabric made up of more cells, the possibilities of this disease are staggering.

There are several classifications of lupus. *Systemic lupus erythematosus* (SLE) is the most prevalent type and the one that is an autoimmune disease. We will focus here on SLE and refer to it simply as lupus. *Discoid lupus erythematosus* is a treatable skin disorder that affects the face, scalp, and other areas of the body. People with discoid lupus do not generally progress to systemic lupus. *Drug-induced lupus* refers to a disease brought on specifically by ingesting certain medications. Drug-induced lupus produces symptoms similar to those of SLE, such as joint pain, rash, and fever. Symptoms resolve when the drug is stopped.

Lupus is one of the more common autoimmune diseases. It is primarily a disease of young women such as Jess. In fact, more than 90 percent of sufferers in this country are women whose symptoms began between the ages of eighteen and fifty. Various theories have been put forth on the association between the two, one of which includes the effect of estrogen on the immune system. (See chapter 1 for a more in-depth explanation on this topic.)

I have heard estimates of around 2.5 million lupus sufferers in this country alone, although the true numbers are difficult to determine because the symptoms of the disease vary so widely and because so many people do not even know they have it. I am certain that as I sit here writing this book, thousands of people with lupus are traveling from doctor to doctor to doctor with their amorphous symptoms, searching for an accurate diagnosis.

The prevalence of lupus appears to vary with ethnicity. It is estimated that in the United States, the disease affects about 1 in 250 African-Americans, 1 in 500 Latinos, and 1 in 1,000 Caucasians. Lupus is also quite common in China. The underlying reason that certain races are more prone to this disease than others is not well understood.

Natural Course of the Disease

Like some other autoimmune diseases—rheumatoid arthritis and multiple sclerosis, for example—lupus is manifested by acute episodes (periods of active disease) known as flares, in which symptoms erupt suddenly and then resolve. Things remain quiet for an unpredictable amount of time until the disease flares again. During a lupus flare, different symptoms can occur at different times, and new symptoms may continue to appear years after the original diagnosis.

Lupus flares normally arise every six months to a year, and sometimes more often. A flare can come on suddenly, starting with weakness, low-grade fever, and joint pain. The symptoms are always unpredictable. Flares can last from three days to a month, and the duration may be different each time. Untreated flares generally last longer than treated ones (see later on). Between flares, patients are considered to be in remission.

Although this is primarily a young woman's disease, lupus can also occur for the first time at any time after menopause. I have seen patients upward of ninety get lupus for the first time, but it is not commonly seen, and the symptoms are far milder than the stormy course associated with those that befall younger women. There are certain conditions—thyroiditis is one of them—which I believe predispose women after menopause to autoimmune diseases such as lupus. The good news is that lupus gets better as the patient gets older. The intervals between flares widen, and symptoms, when they occur, are greatly diminished in strength. No matter when the first symptoms of lupus appear, life expectancy for treated lupus patients remains the same as for those who do not have the disease.

Symptoms of Lupus

Symptoms of lupus arise when antibodies perceive certain components of a cell—such as the cell nucleus or cell cytoplasm—as antigenic and assault them. The attachment of antigen and antibody form an immune complex that ultimately causes inflammation, the basis for the symptomatic pain, redness of the skin, and shifts in fluid around the joints that produce typical lupus-related swelling. Because the entire body consists of cells, inflamed tissue can be found almost anywhere. Lupus can affect any or all systems, including the joints, skin, heart, lungs, kidneys, blood, and brain. Any of the resulting symptoms can singularly wreak havoc in a body. For example:

▷ When the central nervous system is involved, the results are headaches, memory disturbances, vision problems, or behavioral changes.
▷ When the target is the kidney, inflammation, though painless, brings blood into the urine and seriously compromises the kidney's ability to get rid of waste products effectively.
▷ When lupus affects the lungs, the result is *pleuritis*—an inflammation of the lining of the chest cavity, which may lead to breathing difficulty, pain, and pneumonia.

▷ Lupus of the blood can result in anemia or a decrease in platelets, a condition called *thrombocytopenia*, which is at the root of ITP (idiopathic thrombocytopenic purpura) another autoimmune disease that is the focus of chapter 4. People with lupus also have an increased risk of developing blood clots, the main symptom in vasculitis. Lupus also can occur along with antiphospholipid syndrome, another platelet-related autoimmune disease. (See chapter 3.)

▷ When lupus affects the heart, the results can be myocarditis, endocarditis, or pericarditis, among other potentially dangerous effects.

▷ Lupus can cause temporary alopecia (hair loss). Small patches of hair fall out at the time of a flare, but it generally grows back when the flare subsides.

▷ The skin is affected when a person with lupus is exposed to the sun. Sun sensitivity occurs in about 60 percent of lupus patients and results in a rash across the sun-exposed areas. A malar rash (redness across the cheeks) is also closely associated with this disease and appears as a result of the autoimmune attack.

▷ One of the more common symptoms associated with lupus is Raynaud's phenomenon, which is discussed in depth in chapter 15 on scleroderma. Raynaud's causes a temporary blanching, or turning white, of the fingers and sometimes of the toes. This occurs when the capillaries at the tips of the fingers spontaneously go into spasm and shut down.

There is no set pattern to this disease, and Jess is a perfect example of this. At first, she had only some of the more common symptoms: painful joints, extreme fatigue, fever, and skin rash. The *butterfly rash* that radiated across the bridge of her nose is typical for some 30 to 50 percent of patients, and it is the basis for the signs and logos used by lupus organizations around the world. Jess's fever stemmed from the release of chemicals by white blood cells as they assaulted specific tissues, which they confused with an antigen. Her warm, reddened joints also reflected inflammation. As we saw, in time her kidneys became involved. As white cells come into the kidneys at the signal of the immune lymphocytes and as antibodies are released into the urine, cell debris leaks out of the kidney, resulting in a loss of protein. This causes fluid to back up into the tissues and results in swelling—the same swelling that I observed in Jess on that afternoon in my office. Why lupus targets one bodily system and not another is anyone's guess. It is just the nature of this particular disease.

Causes of Lupus

No one knows for sure what causes lupus. The conventional wisdom is that it is brought on by a combination of genetic, environmental, and possibly hormonal factors. But although genetics is thought to play a role, to date we have not been able to identify a lupus gene. It may actually turn out that more than one gene is required to increase a person's susceptibility to the disease. In favor of the genetic theory is that lupus can run in families. Studies of identical twins, who share identical sets of genes, show that lupus occurs in both twins far more often (from 25 to 50 percent) than it does in fraternal twins or other siblings (5 percent). It is also known that first-degree relatives (parents, siblings, and children) of people with lupus have a 5 to 12 percent greater tendency to develop the disease. In any case, lupus does not seem to be passed down in the typical Mendelian manner, in which, as I mentioned earlier, if you have the gene you will get the disease, such as with muscular dystrophy and Huntington's disease.

The fact that this disease is so heavily skewed toward women has been a subject of study for quite some time. We know that the immune system is stimulated by hormones, but to what degree is unknown. Although lupus generally is considered a disease that occurs during the childbearing years, men, older women, and young children can get the disease, so it stands to reason that if hormones do play a role, it is probably in conjunction with some other trigger.

Beyond genetics and hormones, scientists are examining other factors that appear to exacerbate the disease. These include sun exposure, ultraviolet light exposure, infections that stress the body (such as herpes or flu), pregnancy, emotional stress, and certain drugs.

About 10 percent of people with lupus are thought to have acquired it through the body's interaction with a particular medication, although no one seems to be able to understand how the drugs cause the body to react against itself. According to published reports, at last count there are some 200 medicines that have the potential to induce the symptoms of lupus. The three most common are *pronestyl*, which is used to treat irregular heartbeats, *hydralazine*, which is used to control blood pressure, and *isoniazid* (INH), an antitubercular drug. When the drug is discontinued, lupus symptoms disappear, but the process can take up to a year.

Diagnosing Lupus

Lupus is difficult to diagnose and hard to treat. It is so complex, in fact, that the clinical findings in any two patients may be completely different, yet both can be correctly consigned the diagnosis of lupus. I am not even sure this is *one* illness. Indeed, it may be a series of illnesses that has as its basis an autoimmune response.

Because lupus touches so many of the body's systems, it is often confused with other diseases. For example, some of the symptoms of lupus—sore and stiff muscles and joints—mimic the rheumatic diseases, such as Sjögren's syndrome and rheumatoid arthritis. The fatigue, fever, and muscle spasms that are so common in many autoimmune diseases are present in lupus. The platelet diseases—APLS and ITP—mimic lupus, and so does diabetic-induced kidney disease. Even some of the rashes are similar. The malar rash associated with lupus looks very much like dermatomyositis, a skin condition associated with autoimmune muscle disease. Other diseases that are often confused with lupus include syphilis, Lyme disease, flu, herpes, chronic fatigue syndrome, and fibromyalgia. Sometimes the only way to differentiate the diseases is by doing an antibody evaluation and weeding them out. This is discussed later.

I have seen countless patients with lupus, and even with twenty-five years of experience, during which time I edited and wrote for two textbooks on the disease, I am the first to admit that it still takes me a long time to make a definitive diagnosis. To illustrate the process, let us return to Jess, and I will show you precisely what transpired between the time she arrived in my office and the time I was able to give her an unequivocal diagnosis.

Diagnosing Jess

Jess, if you recall, came to see me after first being examined by a number of other physicians. I read the other doctors' notes and then took an extensive history myself, in which she described her symptoms: chronic low-grade fever, fatigue, joint aches, and a rash. Next, I examined her and found not only evidence of all these things, but saw that her body was slightly swollen as well. This made me suspect that she had an autoimmune disease, but from just her symptoms, it might have been anything from rheumatoid arthritis to vasculitis, from Sjögren's syndrome to lupus, and more.

My next move was to consider which diseases were likely and which were unlikely, and so I proceeded to rule them out one by one. She had no dry eyes or lack of saliva, so I knew it was unlikely to be Sjögren's. It was unlikely to be autoimmune muscle disease, because her muscles were not weak or painful when I pressed them. It was certainly not rheumatoid arthritis, because although there was joint swelling, it was not in the specific areas that point to rheumatoid arthritis. The more diseases I ruled out, the closer I was to suspecting she had lupus.

In order to back up my suspicion, my next step was to turn to the laboratory. Because lupus is so complex, there is no single laboratory test that can diagnose all cases. The most effective laboratory tests for lupus include the search for antinuclear autoantibodies, or ANAs. But even if these antibodies are found, it is not 100 percent conclusive, because many people who are positive for ANAs do not necessarily have the disease—in fact, at low concentration, ANAs can be found in just about anybody, with our without autoimmune disease. A positive ANA tells me only that that person is able to make autoantibodies. Further, a positive ANA can be found in rheumatoid arthritis, Sjögren's, and scleroderma. ANAs are also found in pregnant women and the elderly. So although the test could not clinch the diagnosis of lupus, it did tell me that her immune system was reacting to something that it perceived as foreign.

Jess returned to the lab a week later, and we ran three more tests. First up was a *complement test. Complement* is a series of proteins found in the blood. In the face of an immune reaction, complement is soaked up and disposed of by the immune system. If I measure complement and the results show it is low or nonexistent, it tells me, like the ANA, that there is acute immune activity, but again, not necessarily involving lupus. Still, a positive test suggests that I should go further and look for more antibodies. The second test was for anti-DNA antibodies. Lupus is a disease of the cell nucleus, so if someone has lupus, the antibodies will be shown to react with DNA. For the third test, we looked for an anti-Smith antigen. Anti-Smith is present in 35 percent of lupus cases. Jess was positive for anti-DNA and anti-Smith, and this, coupled with her other signs and symptoms, clinched the diagnosis for both of us.

Treating Lupus

The art of medicine is never so refined as when we select the right treatment for a patient. As soon as I was certain of her diagnosis, Jess and I went about devising a treatment plan that would be both effective and realistic for her. The three main treatment objectives for any lupus patient are to try to prevent flares (or at least to minimize their duration and severity), to treat them as they occur, and to prevent organ damage and other complications.

Because lupus is the result of inflammation left behind after immune complexes go to work, the initial treatment for this disease is aimed at reducing the inflammation. A group of medications are designed to help, including anti-inflammatories, corticosteroids, immunosupressants, and chemotherapy. If a patient has joint or chest pain, I prescribe drugs that also act on swelling, usually a type of nonsteroidal anti-inflammatory (NSAID). While some of these can easily be purchased without a prescription, they must be taken under a doctor's direction because they can produce side effects that can mask the start of other dangerous situations, such as kidney failure, stomach problems, or internal bleeding. See chapter 17 for more in-depth information about these drugs.

Antimalarial drugs are effective too, but we are not sure why. It is possible that they work by suppressing parts of the immune response. These miraculous drugs do remarkable things with almost no side effects. Antimalarials have a side benefit of lowering cholesterol and even slightly thinning the blood. The lowering of cholesterol is particularly beneficial because the most common cause of death in lupus patients is premature heart disease due to accelerated atherosclerosis (the buildup of cholesterol-type fat on the inside surface of the arteries). Thinning the blood is important because more than 40 percent of lupus patients have antiphospholipid antibodies that cause the blood to clot prematurely. *Hydroxychloroquine (plaquenil)* is used for fatigue, joint pain, skin rash, and lung inflammation, but the mainstays are corticosteroid hormones, prednisone, and decadron, a natural anti-inflammatory hormone. These are discussed in detail in chapter 17.

I started Jess on the immunosuppressant prednisone at high doses in order to slow her immune reaction. Within a week, she had gained back most of her energy, but not all. In any case, she felt much better. She was able to lift her baby, play tag with her son, work in her garden, and do all the things that were so difficult for her before the diagnosis. Moreover, her kidney lesions all but totally disappeared, and her kidney functions improved to the point that she did not need chemotherapy.

Preventing Lupus Flares

I explained to Jess that over the next six months to a year, she would probably have one or more short flares of the disease for no apparent reason. But I also told her that just knowing how to predict a flare, when one is coming, would be helpful because treatment could then begin right away, which would lessen the severity of the symptoms. Headache, muscle and joint pain, rash, dizziness, and increased fatigue are some of the indications a flare is imminent. If these symptoms occur, there are some strategies that might help. In fact, these strategies are good examples for daily living for all lupus patients, whether in remission or not.

▷ Eat a healthful diet, one that is low in fat, low in sodium, high in fiber, and low in refined sugars. The recommended diet for lupus is similar to the diets put forth by the American Heart Association and the American Cancer Society. Diets such as the Atkins, which are high in protein, are not recommended only because patients with lupus tend to have compromised kidney function, and a high-protein diet can put stress on the kidneys.

▷ Engage in moderate exercise, particularly when symptoms are not pronounced. Anything that is aerobic, such as walking, biking, or swimming, is helpful. Regular exercise lessens fatigue and gives a general sense of well-being.

▷ Do not engage in any isometric exercises or weightlifting. While these exercises may build muscle, they can stress the body unnecessarily, which can cause particular problems for people with lupus.

▷ Rest. When lupus is active, rest is essential. This may mean restructuring your schedule so that you can take daytime naps. Planning the day so that the pace is as unstressed as possible is an essential part of keeping lupus in check.

▷ Try to keep stress to a minimum. Over the years, many methods have been shown to minimize stress, including meditation, walking, and yoga. Aerobic exercise, such as walking or swimming, is a good stress reliever, too.

▷ Call your physician at the first indication of a flare. The more common symptoms to be aware of include fever, joint pain, and skin rash.

One year after her lupus diagnosis, Jess is almost off prednisone and on a somewhat milder treatment—an antimalarial pill. Although she has gained some weight from the prednisone, she is still a beautiful young woman with two very healthy children and a loving husband, and she has a long life ahead of her. Her condition will have to be carefully monitored, however, especially if she decides to have more children. Even if she does not have more children, Jess, like others with lupus, can expect symptoms of the disease to return.

Lupus and Pregnancy

Some physicians say that pregnancy exacerbates lupus, and others say it may cause the disease, but again, no one really knows. In my experience with pregnant women who have lupus, I subscribe to the rule of thirds: during the pregnancy, one third stay the same, one third get worse, and one third get better during the pregnancy. Classically, if you have active disease—that is, you are experiencing a lupus flare—and you become pregnant, lupus-related symptoms will generally (but not always) increase in severity.

So, is it wise to wait to become pregnant until a lupus flare subsides? Given that a lupus flare generally lasts only a month or two, and then subsides for three or four months, I think it might be a good idea to wait, particularly because the fertility rates of women with lupus are identical to that of women in the general population. Unfortunately, the same cannot be said for pregnancy. Women with lupus experience a fair number of stillbirths and miscarriages, which goes back to my theory about pregnancy and the fine regulation the immune system has on the gestational period.

Can you do anything to care for yourself if you are pregnant with lupus? Yes, yes, yes! You can remain aware that if you have lupus, your pregnancy is considered a high risk. As much as I do not like to say this, that means you must remain aware that at any point in time you may lose your baby. If you get pregnant, you should be under the care of both your rheumatologist and your obstetrician, and your obstetrician should see you so frequently that you get sick of each other. That way, at least if you become likely to miscarry, the obstetrician can take every possible measure to prevent it. I offer identical advice to women with antiphospholipid syndrome (see chapter 3), in which one of the three prevailing symptoms is multiple miscarriage.

According to NIH statistics, one in four babies born to mothers with lupus is born prematurely. I strongly advise my pregnant lupus patients to find a hospital with an excellent neonatal intensive care unit (NICU) and to have access to that hospital at time of delivery, just in case the baby requires special attention. Babies do not seem to suffer any lupus-related birth defects, however. At last, there is some good news.

With lupus, the high risk for women continues after the baby's birth. In many cases, the disease comes back with a vengeance two or three weeks after delivery, so it is a good idea to work with your family and your doctor to plan accordingly.

The way autoimmune diseases behave continues to awe me. Here is a perfect example: When a woman who is predisposed to lupus but has not yet had any symptoms becomes pregnant or delivers a baby, lupus symptoms become evident, which is precisely what happened with Jess. Women who already have lupus find that with pregnancy, their symptoms are exacerbated. In pregnant women with rheumatoid arthritis (RA), however, the reverse is the case. Pregnancy alleviates symptoms to such a degree, in fact, that I have had patients with RA who want to get pregnant just to get rid of their symptoms. Here is a classic example of why we doctors in this field spend so much time scratching our heads. This is just one more of the great mysteries of autoimmune disease.

The Future of Lupus Research

In what I consider one of the most exciting and cutting-edge aspects of autoimmunity today, lupus has begun to provide scientists with new insights into common ailments. One great example of this is atherosclerosis. It is well known that many lupus patients have accelerated atherosclerosis, a buildup of plaque on the inner walls of an artery and a precursor to coronary artery disease and strokes. Scientific studies are looking at whether this may be due to the direct actions of autoantibodies or the indirect actions of cytokines and chemokines on the blood-vessel wall, or it may be due to the effects of an antibody to fats in the blood. Such an encounter could change the balance of fats everywhere in the body. Research will also tell us if such accumulation promotes or protects the vessel walls from the accumulation of plaque and eventual stroke and heart attack. When one considers that atherosclerotic heart disease is the most common cause of death in the Western world, scientific investigation into the mechanics of a disease such as lupus suddenly becomes important to hundreds of millions of people.

Another study is examining the use of *dihydroepiandrosterone*

(DHEA), a weakened male hormone, to treat the disease. DHEA has been sold for years as a nutritional supplement but it seems to be helpful in alleviating some lupus symptoms. (See chapters 19 and 20 for a more extensive discussion.)

In May 2003, I spoke at a Lupus Society meeting attended by hundreds of physicians who came to discuss the latest treatments, diagnosis, and new ideas about lupus. Every time I go to one of these meetings, I am impressed with the elegant work that so many scientists, academics, and physicians are doing to try to prevent and treat this disease. I am further impressed by how well these dedicated people understand the ultimate focus of their research—that is, no matter how high-tech the medical profession becomes, in the end, the only thing that counts is the woman with two young kids who wants to function well day to day and live to see her children grow older.

I have always said that I believed we would see a cure for lupus before I die, but at this point, I am not so sure. Even after the dozens of presentations and the discussions at the meeting, it was clear to me that lupus still has us all stymied. It seems the more we learn, the more complex the immune system seems to become. The overall limited number of drugs available to treat lupus, despite years of research, is a perfect example of how hard it is for the scientific community to understand the biology of this disease. Although there is no cure for lupus, at least it can be treated successfully with appropriate drugs and, happily, most people, like Jess, can go on to lead normal, active lives.

CHAPTER ELEVEN

ALOPECIA UNIVERSALIS

Bald All Over

WHAT CAN ONE say about a disease that makes you long for just one more bad hair day? True, it is not life threatening. And no, it does not even give rise to illness. Still, for the far too many Americans who experience *alopecia universalis* every year, this disease is a catastrophe.

Alopecia universalis (AU), which refers to total loss of hair on the head and body, is an autoimmune disease in which the immune system mistakenly perceives the hair follicles as antigenic and sets out to destroy them. In this disease, T cells assault the rapidly dividing hair follicle cells, causing the follicles to shut down and ultimately stop growing hair. Because this disease is systemic, it wipes out hair across the board—everywhere on the body that hair grows.

An AU attack happens quickly. In a matter of days there is hair on the pillow as though the barber had cut it, hair in the shower that clogs the drain, hair around the house where it does not belong, and none, sadly, where it does. One little detour of an antibody and a young woman is suddenly bald all over. Devastated, she may think her beauty has evaporated. I, for one, do not agree. But more on that subject later.

Types of Alopecia

There are several types of alopecia, only some of which are autoimmune-related.

Male pattern baldness. Also known as *androgenic alopecia,* this is the most common type of alopecia, the one that affects men with regularity and can occur in women, if in a somewhat different pattern. Androgenic alopecia is not immune-related; it is hormone-related and is caused by a processing defect in the follicle at the root of the hair shaft. Men exhibit different patterns of baldness—from receding hairlines, to bald pates fringed at the edges with hair, to total baldness. When the disorder occurs in women, the result is a more diffuse thinning of the hair across the scalp. Androgenic alopecia is the result of a much-maligned hormone called *dihydrotestosterone* (DHT), which affects the hair follicle. An over- or underabundance of this hormone is generally thought to be genetically related.

Alopecia areata (AA). This disease affects one woman in a thousand (it affects men as well) and may or may not be autoimmune-related. Women with AA generally lose their hair in quarter-sized patches over different areas of the scalp. Sometimes only a small amount of scalp is affected and only for a short while. Spontaneous recovery generally happens within six months to a year, but new patches may appear as older ones resolve, so the duration of the disease can be extended indefinitely.

Autoimmune AA can be primary (stand alone) or secondary to some other immune disease. In fact, many autoimmune diseases have alopecia as a secondary issue. One example is vitamin B_{12} deficiency associated *pernicious anemia,* where the blood count plummets because of an immune blockage of vitamin absorption. Women with lupus and Sjögren's syndrome often lose their hair, but it usually comes back within one to twelve months. People with hypothyroidism (too little thyroid hormone) and hyperthyroidism (too much thyroid hormone) lose their hair in a more diffuse pattern, but it often generally returns after treatment. In some cases, when we treat various autoimmune diseases with chemotherapy, patients can lose their hair, but as with the other diseases, hair starts growing back as soon as the chemotherapy is over.

Alopecia areata will often accompany an autoimmune skin disease known as *vitiligo*. This disease occurs when an antibody cross-reacts with the skin pigment cells called *melanosomes*. The result is a loss of skin pigment in patches over certain areas of the body. Vitiligo, which is found in less than 10 percent of people with alopecia, generally appears first on the hands and face but can affect the pubic area and other places as well. Small, irregularly shaped patches of colorless skin the size of a nickel can arise initially, but may spread at a slow pace, over time. The color does not return.

Alopecia totalis (AT). A variant of AA, aleopecia totalis refers to a complete loss of hair but only on the scalp. Hair may or may not return, and the disease may or may not be autoimmune-related.

Alopecia universalis (AU). The subject disease of this chapter, this is actually a form of alopecia areata that extends over the entire body—scalp, arms, legs, eyelashes and eyebrows, and pubis. This type of alopecia is always autoimmune-related—a result of T cells cross-reacting with hair follicles—but for some unknown reason, when the immune system sees one hair follicle as foreign, it sees all of them the same way, meaning that it will affect every hair on the body. Why some patients get AT or AA and others get AU is not understood.

Unfortunately, the hair is not always the only object of the miscreant T cell's attentions. As if losing every hair on the body were not enough, AU also can affect the nails, leaving them pitted, opaque, and ridged at the edge. In extreme cases, the nails may be shed altogether. When nails and hair are affected simultaneously, it is because they are both parts of the same *anlage,* that is, the same embryologically related systems. All of our body's tissues develop from different cell systems. For example, the gastrointestinal tract develops from one, the immune system develops from another, the brain from another, and the bones from still another. Likewise, the germinal tissues that, in the embryo, are destined to develop into the hair also develop into nails as part of that particular system. Because of the close embryological connection of the hair and nails, it is no surprise that an antibody against one (hair) would affect the other (nails).

The Causes of Alopecia Universalis

No one really knows what triggers the immune attack, but my guess is that the culprit is probably a virus with an antigenic structure that mimics some aspect of the hair follicle. Genetics seem to play a role as well, but only in rendering a person more susceptible to the disease. Although some scientists believe AU is hereditary, in my practice I have never heard anyone say someone else in the family has had it. Still, some people are convinced that there is a genetic predisposition to this disease, and indeed there has been an abundance of work in this area. Do you remember the HLA genetic markers on cells? In AU, the HLA markers found on chromosome 6 are the HLA-DR4, -DR11 and -DQ*03. By studying large numbers of people with AU, geneticists have been able to link the occurrence of generalized hair loss in different people to these genes. In a person so predisposed, a virus or some environmental factor like mercury or a red dye might trigger the immune system.

What else do we know of the causes of this disease? Not very much. Only that it seems to be more prevalent in people in their early twenties and thirties, and that it is not caused by stress. Yes, there is alopecia secondary to stress, but it is not autoimmune-related.

Ginny's Story

To put a face to this disease, let me tell you about Ginny, a very beautiful woman who has been a patient of mine for years. An airline flight attendant since she was in her twenties, Ginny knew the importance of grooming in her particular job and carried it through into her everyday life. The day her hair started falling out, which it did quickly and in clumps, she ran frantically to the nearest emergency room and then to her dermatologist. The dermatologist gave her a prescription for Minoxidil and sent her to me.

As I was out of town for a week, by the time Ginny arrived at my office, she had already lost a good deal of her hair. She arrived wearing oversize sunglasses and a print scarf with a baseball cap over it; a few wispy strands of blond hair escaped from the side near her temples. These strands were all that was left, and I knew even they would fall out over the next few days. I suggested that she could at least remove the glasses, explaining that it was just the two of us in the room. She took off her glasses and her cap, tugged her scarf in tighter under her neck, and sat down in the chair across my desk. "You know what, Dr. Lahita?" she said. "I stood in the shower with my razor this morning and tried to decide if I should shave my legs one last time or slit my wrists."

Not an easy line to respond to. But I tried. "You look to be otherwise healthy, though."

"How can you look healthy when you're bald?" she asked, her eyes filling. "You've got to do something. Anything!"

We spoke for a while and then she reluctantly removed her scarf and rubbed the palm of her hand across her shiny scalp. Indeed, most of her hair was gone. So were her eyebrows and eyelashes. I did not feel the need to do extensive diagnostic testing on Ginny because with this disease, the history and physical findings say it all. I knew it was AU because she had lost her eyebrows and eyelashes. Still, I suggested running some blood work. As I have learned over and over again, it pays to be thorough—sometimes medicine can fool you.

Diagnosing Alopecia Universalis

I ordered a preliminary blood workup to see if Ginny was indeed as healthy as she looked. She was. I also wanted to know if any autoimmune proteins or autoantibodies could be found in her blood. None were obvious, but that can happen with this disease. I then removed a few strands of remaining hair from around her temples to examine the character of the hair shaft and the properties of the hair follicle. The small, bulblike follicle appears different in people with AU because the growth areas in the skin are arrested. This test was positive, and essentially told me what I already knew. All that was left was to try to treat her.

Treating Alopecia Universalis

Treatment for AU is very slow to show results, if indeed it shows them at all. The time period—often up to six months for just a meager result—is additionally unsettling to someone already in a fragile emotional state. Treating AU is much simpler than treating other autoimmune diseases. You know what you are dealing with, and all that is left is to try to find some treatment that will work.

I always qualify any treatment plan before I begin it by telling my patients with AU two things: In some cases, hair may grow back spontaneously with no treatment, but it can take months and more often, years, and it may fall out again at any time. I also tell them that as far as I know, while in some instances drugs or lotions may promote (sparse) hair growth, nothing can prevent new patches of loss or actually cure the underlying disease.

I speak from years of experience. I have injected steroids such as prednisone under the *gallia*, the top layer of skin on the scalp. This results in tufts of hair that pop up like weeds in a garden, but the hair falls out again within two weeks. I have used other immunosuppressive drugs, such as cyclosporine and plaquenil, an antimalarial drug, both by mouth and injection. The hair began to grow back as peach fuzz, but in no case was I able to regrow the hair completely. Ointments containing steroids also can be rubbed into or sprayed on the affected area, but they are even less effective and must be used daily.

On the positive side, as I write this book, there are some new agents about to come out on the market, if they have not already done so. And there are some old agents used in new ways. Of late, the scientific literature is replete with success stories after treatment for AU. Some of the newer immunosuppressants used for this disease include *tacrolimus cream*—also called FK506—which is rubbed on the scalp. This is a potent antirejection drug that is given to transplant patients orally. Perhaps soon there will be more agents to try in the near future. I learned long ago that with alopecia of any type, patience is key.

Ginny and I decided she would try plaquenil—a gentle immuno-suppressant—by mouth, and that she would liberally apply Minoxidil daily to her scalp. Minoxidil is a blood pressure drug that in low concentration can sometimes help to grow hair. The problem with Minoxidil is that as soon as you stop using it, the new hair stops growing. It hardly worked at all for Ginny. In six months, the only hair that grew was a fine down. At that point we talked abut what we would do next, and I explained that going to anything stronger than plaquenil would work against her immune system, so we stopped there. I am a strong believer that one must balance the good with the bad effects of therapy. In a possibly futile attempt to cure baldness, I will not place a patient's well-being in absolute jeopardy by using drugs that can severely lower her white cells and ultimately leave her vulnerable to infection, even if it means denying her a little bit of hair.

I would like to digress for a moment to openly express my thoughts on treating alopecia in general. I have seen many women, young and old, become despondent because their hair fell out with a lupus flare, or, for example, when I put them on chemotherapy for their polymyositis—an autoimmune muscle disease (see chapter 16). To these women, the hair fallout seems to be more important than the underlying disease or treatment, which, as a doctor and a man, I simply do not understand. If they could grow back their hair, they say, they would be willing to tolerate everything else. This also holds true, and often more so, for women with AU, who want the strongest of the strong drugs, at the risk of kidney damage and more.

I just do not get it. Sometimes I sit back and visualize a big ruler against a wall. On one end are the kidney, the liver, the heart, and the lungs; on the other are fingernails, hair, and saliva. There I am at the kidney end, worrying like crazy how to keep my patients alive and well, and they are focused on the hair and nails end, unhappy because they do not like how they look. To the extent that this makes me sound like a chauvinist, I apologize, and yes, I understand that some women depend on their looks a great deal, but what good are looks without *life*? Which brings me to another point: Why is it that some women can so easily look beyond appearance when it comes to others, yet their own looks matter so much to them? When a woman with alopecia universalis comes to see me, I look at her from the vantage point of her physician who is worried about her illness, her health, and her life. I really feel for these young women, and my heart goes out to them, but I do think we need to keep things in perspective. Lecture over.

Alopecia Research

I am both thrilled and amazed at the interest that has been sparked by this disease of late. There is so much that is new and encouraging, thanks to the scientists in the field of dermatology and autoimmunology who have taken on the challenge with great energy. Following are some of the issues currently being investigated.

As I mentioned earlier, the wonders of the natural pregnant state offer many comparisons to RA and MS because both diseases go into remission during those nine months. Research on monocytes—a form of white cells taken from women who have AU—indicate that most pregnant women do not have enough tumor necrosis factor (TNF) or angiogenesis factor in their blood. You might remember TNF as the cytokine that is involved in inflammation, the same one that can be suppressed, with great success, when treating women with rheumatoid arthritis. It is the suppression of TNF that allows these women to live normal lives again. As it turns out, the opposite is true in AU. There is almost no TNF in the blood of the AU patient to suppress. This could mean that this hair loss of pregnancy is somehow related to the absence of the TNF in the natural pregnant state.

Another scientific investigation project concerns angiogenesis factor, a blood-vessel-growing element that is present in our blood and helps blood vessels regenerate in damaged tissues. The low levels of this factor in women with AU might mean that blood-vessel generation might be compromised in this population. This major finding could indicate that besides the immune problems, there is a defect in the formation of blood vessels at the microscopic level.

Still other recent research indicates that the genetic link to AU might be quite significant. The finding of identical twins both having AU with virtually the same onset is startling and indicates that there is a large contribution of genetics to this immune response. Unfortunately, because finding identical twins with AU is so difficult—this is, after all, a fairly rare disease—the population group of patients to investigate is small. In other diseases, such as lupus, the occurrence in twins can be calculated because there are many cases of lupus-suffering identical twins to study. AU has occurred with other illnesses such as Crohn's disease, polymyositis, hardening of the bile ducts in the liver (called *sclerosing cholangitis*), and chronic inflammatory polyneuropathy or "immune nerve disease" (a particularly vexing problem). All of these diseases have some contribution of genetics to their acquisition.

Ginny's Story, Continued

Ginny came back to see me every six weeks or so for a while, and each time she would admonish me to "do something" or "try anything." We did try several of the new drugs, but in her case, they did not do very much. Still, throughout her treatment she kept the faith: "Dr. Lahita, I know you can fix this. I know you can." It is times like this that medicine can be so frustrating. Much as I wanted to be that little engine that could, I could not be sure this lovely woman would ever again have a hair on her body.

After a while, we began to talk about her future and the fact that the she might have to accept the inevitable. And slowly, slowly, she came around. Then, one day, I read in a journal article of a new treatment that just might do the trick. The report said that topical cyclosporine A, a potent immunosuppressive, was fairly harmless if used on the scalp over a short term. It suggested that this drug, accompanied by prednisone by mouth at limited doses, had helped some patients with AU. Ginny wanted to try it, and because I believed it was safe, I agreed. We began the treatment and after three months, it appeared as though some patches of hair were coming in, if not as luxuriously as both of us had hoped. Four months later at our office visit, she announced that she was getting married. He was an airline pilot with a seven-year-old daughter, a wonderful man who thought she was gorgeous with or without her hair. The marriage took her to Texas and, as often happens, I lost track of her.

But not forever. Two years later Ginny came back to New York for a visit and she came in to see me. She wore a snappy black suit and white shirt. Her hair (a blond wig) was cut short and wispy around her face; her eyebrows were penciled in a dark blond. "You're glowing," I told her. "You look great! Must be the blond hair."

Stupid me. And a father of two. I should have guessed about the glow.

In the examining room, Ginny took off her wig and showed me "a wonderful surprise . . ." Her hair was growing back, even if not yet thickly enough for her to go out comfortably in public without her wig. I explained to her that this time it was the *pregnancy*, not the drugs, that was doing the trick. I know she was disappointed to hear that, but her life was going so well, she seemed to take that news in stride.

Benefits of Pregnancy

As with rheumatoid arthritis, multiple sclerosis, and some of the other autoimmune diseases, the symptoms of the AU may resolve with pregnancy, which means that the immune system temporarily discontinues its assault. Why this happens in some of these diseases and not others, no one knows, but I can assure you, if I won the lottery tomorrow and never had to work another day, I would concentrate on finding the answer. Pregnancy-related remission of autoimmune diseases is completely fascinating!

Will Ginny's new hair continue growing after her baby is born? Probably not. Does she care? Of course. But she can deal with it. She has made a wonderful life for herself, and who knows what can happen next? I would never have bet on any return of hair for her, and so it was doubly pleasing for me to watch her pull off her wig with an "I told you so" look on her face.

Living with Alopecia Universalis

I love happy endings. I only wish all my patients with AU had such wonderful finales to their story. But actually, many do. I'll bet you see them every day on the street. You may *think* you do not know anyone who has this disease, but you would be wrong. Your daughter's math teacher has it. So does your dry cleaner's wife. The reason you don't know about them is that they, like so many others with alopecia, have mastered the tricks of the trade. Until we beat this disease back into the woods, a well-made wig and a trip to the cosmetics counter for a few good tips with an eyebrow pencil can work wonders. Just ask Ginny.

CHAPTER TWELVE

SJÖGREN'S SYNDROME

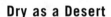

Dry as a Desert

"I'M A MESS," said Laura. The truth is, she was right. Whatever she had, her symptoms had clearly gotten the best of her. Her eyes were red and gloppy, her tongue swollen, her lips cracked. I got an additional clue about her physical state from how she seated herself when she approached my desk—slowly and with far more care than you would expect from a forty-two-year-old woman. Her referring doctor told me she was a very successful retail executive with a high-powered job, two teenage sons, and a husband in marketing. What I saw was a stunning woman with thick black hair, now graying, wearing wire-rimmed glasses, and dressed in an impeccably well-tailored suit. She was also clearly miserable. I asked her to tell me about it.

"Actually, I've been feeling lousy for quite some time. A year perhaps, even longer," she said. "All these things were going wrong. Small things at first, you know? I'd get sick, then I'd be better for a while, then sick again. Everything appeared unrelated, so I just took each illness as it came. But now, some of them are overlapping, and what's more upsetting is that they're getting worse instead of better. And they are bizarre. For example, when I eat some foods I've always loved, like kosher pickles or even fruit, my tongue feels as if someone is pouring hot soup over it. I'm having trouble swallowing just about everything, unless I wash it down with liquid. If I keep my contact lenses in for more than an hour or it feels as if there is sand in my eyes, and sometimes I get up in the morning with my eyelids stuck together. My eyes look so bad, I've actually taken a leave of absence from my job. My muscles feel like someone has used them as a punching bag, and my fingers hurt so much that there are days when I can't hold the telephone without feeling like I'm going to drop it. Plus, I don't have sex with my husband anymore because it feels as if he has razor blades strapped to his penis." She managed a weak smile. "Shall I continue?"

It was not necessary. I know a classic case of Sjögren's when I hear one.

What Is Sjögren's Syndrome?

Sjögren's is an autoimmune disease that strikes young and older women alike. Four out of five Sjögren's patients are women. For unknown reasons, the body's white blood cells mistake its own moisture-producing glands for foreign invaders and proceed to infiltrate and attack them, causing inflammation of the glands and rendering them useless. The glands most commonly involved in Sjögren's are the lachrymal glands, which produce our tears, and the parotid and salivary glands, which are responsible for keeping our mouths wet.

Tears and saliva: two bodily functions we all take so completely for granted. It is like breathing—who thinks about it until it becomes difficult? Ivan Pavlov never took saliva for granted. The Russian professor of physiology studied it for half a century. He knew, through his experiments on dogs, that saliva has a mind of its own, deciding how much to release, when to release it, and when to stop. He also knew that the autonomic nerves, the parasympathetic nerves in particular, give the orders—ratchet the liquid up when we need to swallow, down when we give a speech. The salivary glands perform these duties with great accuracy. Ordinarily, no one pays much attention to saliva. Here, we will.

The lachrymal glands deserve their due as well. Tears lubricate our eyes when we need it, and stop when we do not. Certain nerves turn on the faucets when an eyelash falls onto the eyeball and irritates the eye. They turn them on again at the end of *Casablanca,* when Ingrid Bergman walks slowly out of Humphrey Bogart's life forever. The tear glands, where every single tear is manufactured throughout our lifetime, are located in the upper outer corners of the eyes, just under the eyelids. Here, millions of cells each produce a fragment of the tear. These "tearlets" come together until enough is amassed to produce a single droplet. Ducts transport that droplet, and the next, to the eye in an amount sufficient to coat the eyeball, so that when we blink as the lights suddenly come up at the end of the play, or wink back knowingly at a good friend, the tears keep everything working. (And when we have finished with them, a tiny, half-inch pipe drains the tears into the nose, which is why, at a funeral, all the handkerchiefs come out.) Like saliva, tears are created through silent yet perfectly timed reflexes. Except when, as in Laura's case, they do not come at all.

Symptoms of Sjögren's Syndrome

While the hallmark symptoms of Sjögren's syndrome are lack of saliva and tears, there are far more areas of the body affected by this moisture-robbing disease. Characteristically, with Sjögren's, the mucous membranes—any or all of them—dry up, which is why I call it the *desert syndrome.* Sjögren's can involve the lungs, central and peripheral nervous systems, vagina, and kidneys. As we will see in a minute, the symptoms do not stop there. Although Laura showed no evidence of this, some investigators say that up to 75 percent of Sjögren's patients may have minor behavioral abnormalities such as psychoses or depression. To date, no one has been able to explain the connection to the moisture-producing glands. It surprises me, too, because Sjögren's seems to have no relationship at all to any component of the brain. The only plausible explanation for the behavioral changes and the panoply of psychiatric conditions is the presence of antibodies to antigens in the brain. This is my own theory, and I believe it will turn out to be true. These antibodies, like many others which we find in this disease, may stick to and possibly affect the function of nerve cells.

Chief among the antibodies associated with Sjögren's syndrome is the anti-RO antibody. Anti-RO is found in a variety of other diseases, but not in the strength that we find it in Sjögren's syndrome. The curious thing about the anti-RO antibody is that it is known to cause a form of hereditary heart block—that is, a slowing of the heart rate—in some infants that are born to mothers with the antibody. It does so by attaching to the electrical system of the unborn child's heart. In rare instances, it can cause fetal death when it is not discovered early.

Here are more symptoms of Sjögren's:

▷ Sjögren's can cause excessively dry skin. When it is secondary to lupus—that is, lupus has been diagnosed as the primary disease, but Sjögren's accompanies it—patients who are sensitive to sunlight can suffer sunburn from even a minimum of sun exposure.

▷ Dry mouth can lead to major problems with dental caries. The body normally makes enzymes that protect the mucous membranes and other portals of the body. Enzymes are natural disease fighters that help the policing of the body by the immune system. There are many such enzymes in saliva, but the most prominent one is *lysozyme*. (Dogs have an exceptionally great amount of lysozyme, which is why dogs' mouths are said to be so clean.) Because saliva production is insufficient, a Sjögren's patient has almost none of these protective enzymes. When the teeth and gums are not bathed in the right protective solutions, cavities and gum problems begin.

▷ Dry mouth also can lead to lung problems, which can develop when bacteria in the mouth migrate into the lungs and cause infection, or when bacteria sneak into the lungs and stay there. Untreated, these infections can lead to bronchitis. When I listen to a Sjögren's patient's lungs with my stethoscope, the sounds I hear are reminiscent of a paper bag being crumpled.

▷ Sjögren's syndrome can produce a situation within the central and peripheral nervous systems, causing *paresthesias*—a feeling of tiny electrical shocks in the hands or the feet, or pain, numbness, tingling—and sometimes muscle weakness. This numbness of the hands and feet remains one of the many Sjögren's symptoms that go unexplained. Again, it could be related to the affinity some of these antibodies have for certain parts of the brain.

▷ Sjögren's is closely linked to an autoimmune liver disease called *primary biliary cirrhosis* (see chapter 14) and it also can affect the pancreas, leading to inflammation which results in a very painful, though not autoimmune, condition called *pancreatitis.*

▷ When Sjögren's affects the kidneys, it can cause many problems, but one of the most challenging for rheumatologists as well as the nephrologists (kidney specialists) is renal tubular acidosis, a form of kidney disease in which the kidney is unable to properly process acids and bases.

Understanding Sjögren's Syndrome

Sjögren's is a multisystem disease. However, it is not the most far-reaching disease of all the autoimmune conditions. The winner of that dubious distinction, as we have seen, is lupus. (In this case, Sjögren's will have to settle for the silver medal.) Sjögren's can be both primary and secondary diseases. It can appear, for example, along with and secondary to rheumatoid arthritis, polymyositis, and scleroderma in addition to lupus, as mentioned earlier.

One of the most bizarre and I think one of the most important aspects of this illness in terms of research is the greatly increased risk that Sjögren's patients have of developing lymphoma—that is, cancer of the lymph system. The lymph system—that complex of liquids and cells that are an integral part of the immune system—is the highway of immune function. We know for sure that the lifetime risk of developing lymphoma goes up about forty times upon a diagnosis of Sjögren's. For this reason, if no other, I advise all my patients with this disease to get frequent medical checkups (at least yearly) and to report any new and more unusual symptoms, particularly swollen glands. The most common place for lymphoma to develop in people with Sjögren's is in the salivary gland. Other lymphoma-induced symptoms may include fever and tiredness, itchy skin, and unexplained weight loss.

Sjögren's syndrome was first mentioned, although not by that name, in 1888. A Polish surgeon, Dr. Johannes Freiherr von Mikulicz-Radecki, found cells of the lymphocyte type had filtered into the *parotids* (saliva-producing glands that are found in the cheeks) and lachrymal (tear-producing) glands of a farmer. Then, in 1933, a Swedish eye doctor, Henrik Sjögren, described the initial disease triad of parotid enlargement, lack of saliva, and dry eyes, and the disease was given his name. Now, more than eighty years later, we have learned much, though hardly enough, about the disease and its etiology.

Causes of Sjögren's Syndrome

Those who study this disease believe it is probably caused by a combination of factors, including genetics, infection, and the environment. I use the word "believe" because no one yet has been able to link a specific gene to the Sjögren's. Current research shows that several different genes appear to be involved and can predispose different people to the disease, but none of them alone, as far as we know, causes Sjögren's. Some sort of trigger must activate the immune system first. I believe these triggers most likely are either bacterial or viral in nature.

One prime candidate is the Epstein-Barr virus (EBV). EBV is known to stimulate the production of the rheumatoid factor, which is associated with Sjögren's syndrome and lupus, as well as with rheumatoid arthritis. It may be that that particular virus stimulates the immune system and then the gene alters the way the immune system responds. In other words, in the process of attacking the virus, the misguided lymphocytes also go to the moisture glands and there attack the healthy cells, provoking inflammation and ultimately damaging the glands.

There is another association that bears mention and leads me to believe that this disease is caused by a virus. Fairly recently, a new condition was described in people infected with the HIV virus that was originally thought to be Sjögren's syndrome. This condition is called diffuse infiltrative lymphocytosis syndrome (DILS). DILS symptoms look exactly like those related to Sjögren's syndrome; the enlarged parotid glands and dry eyes, mouth, and mucous membranes are all a part of this condition. The difference is in the physiology of the disease. In DILS, it is the suppressor T cells that operate, instead of the helper T cells that work in regular Sjögren's syndrome. While Sjögren's is only assumed to be connected to a virus, albeit one that we cannot yet identify, the HIV-infected patient is known to have a true virus as the cause of the disease. The fact that DILS is unrelated to Sjögren's syndrome but has identical characteristics may be Mother Nature's way of telling us that Sjögren's is really caused by a virus. It is only a theory, but I believe it's a valid one.

Diagnosing Sjögren's Syndrome

Because the symptoms of Sjögren's so closely mimic those of many other diseases, receiving a definitive diagnosis is not always easy. Most people begin with one specialist and end up with many over a period of years, either searching for an answer to what is wrong with them or to clear up each of the illnesses as they beset them. Depending on how the symptoms run, a woman might first see an allergist for the dryness of her nasal passages, a gynecologist for her dry vagina, an ophthalmologist for her dry eyes, and a pulmonologist when problems such as a persistent dry cough become evident. Like Laura, she may never put things together and notice that the common denominator is dryness. I suppose we could say that in one respect Laura was lucky because she went to her family physician, and he knew enough to send her directly to a rheumatologist (who happened to be me). Still, she waited more than a year before bringing any of her symptoms to that doctor's attention.

As I mentioned earlier, Laura's symptoms were so classically convincing that I might have been able to diagnose her condition without even examining her, but I never feel comfortable doing that. First, I ordered a routine chest X-ray to look for any telltale signs of abnormality and to rule out the presence of large lymph nodes in the chest.

I felt it was important to look for the nodes because they might herald lymphoma, and they also can be the sign of an infection. Next, she had a urinalysis to evaluate her kidney function, some routine blood tests to determine how her liver was functioning, and immunological tests to check for certain antibodies. The latter was most significant because they would tell us if Laura had one or both of the antinuclear antibodies (ANAs) classically found in Sjögren's syndrome—anti-RO and anti-LA (the initials are for the first two patients in whom the antibodies were first described). It turned out she had both.

Just as a reminder, ANAs tell us that a patient's antibodies are working against self-tissue—meaning, of course, that they are autoantibodies. As such, they confirm the existence of autoimmune disease, but they cannot isolate which one. Anti-RO and anti-LA also are found in lupus and other illnesses, but not in such high levels as seen in Sjögren's disease. Another antibody, rheumatoid factor (RF), is found in Sjögren's but also is associated with rheumatoid arthritis. (Rheumatoid factor is discussed in detail in chapter 17.) Presence of RF antibody would have meant Laura might have had rheumatoid arthritis, but when both RF and ANA were present, and with her symptoms of dry eyes and dry mouth so evident, I was confident in making a diagnosis of Sjögren's.

There are two other standard tests for Sjogren's and I performed both of them on Laura just to make perfectly sure I knew what we were dealing with. These tests are a Schirmer test and a lip biopsy. The Schirmer test, which measures tears to see how the lachrymal gland is working, involves placing a small piece of paper in the eye under the lower lid and measuring the level of wetness against a standard guide, to see the amount of tears produced in a particular time period. Compared to virtually every other autoimmune disease test, this is one of the cheapest and most effective, but it is not always clearly diagnostic. I followed that with a salivary gland biopsy of the inside of her lip, which contains many small salivary glands. The biopsy showed that her glands contained lymphocytes in a particular pattern, which cemented the diagnosis, but only because so many of the other signs were indicative of this disease. The lip biopsy itself is rarely clear enough to give us a definitive diagnosis for this disease.

When Laura and I met again in my office a few days later, she still looked bad but somehow brighter. When I commented on this, she said she was very relieved that help was on the way. "While I hate the diagnosis," she said, "I'm grateful to know there *is* a diagnosis, and I'm anxious to get started on treatment." I had explained to her earlier on the phone that while we could not cure her disease, I felt certain most of her symptoms could be managed, and she could go back to living a fairly normal, almost symptom-free, life.

Treating Sjögren's Syndrome

On that visit, Laura and I sat together in my office for an hour and laid out a treatment plan. We took each symptom separately. First, I encouraged her to get rid of her contact lenses and to buy more protective glasses to safeguard her eyes against the wind and natural drying, and I suggested that she use over-the-counter artificial tears, which she was already doing. Next, I suggested a potent vaginal lubricant and prescribed a pilocarpine preparation to increase her saliva. Tending to the inflammation of her joints, I prescribed an anti-inflammatory drug that would make her more comfortable. Finally, I suggested a trip to her dentist, because the lack of saliva was beginning to make her teeth go bad. (Most dentists are aware of this disease and understand how to care for these patients.)

We also discussed that in addition to the treatment plan, there were many things she could do for herself while waiting for the disease to go into remission (which it often does). I explained that it was best to avoid foods that are dehydrating, such as coffee and alcohol, and that cough syrups and other liquids that contain sugar and alcohol must be avoided. So should spicy and acidic foods, including citrus fruits and tomatoes, the juices of which can irritate a sore dry mouth. Of course, Laura had already figured out most of this herself. She also uses a heavy moisturizer on her skin, which occasionally goes through severe dry spells with uncomfortable itching, and she is careful to wear sunscreen with an SPF of thirty or more.

At the conclusion of our visit that day she said, "You know, Doctor Lahita, I've decided to tackle this disease the way I do a business problem. I always tell my staff, 'You have a problem, you figure out how to solve it, then come to me and I'll help you make it happen.' So now with this disease, I'm going to take my own advice." The forthright, take-charge manner in which she spoke that afternoon gave me a glimpse of her in her element, and I knew she would be a patient who took control of the future of her health.

Treatment of Sjögren's syndrome is fairly straightforward, unless the patient stops responding to therapy. Fortunately, this is not common. Still, there are people who take medication but continue to have dry eyes, a dry mouth, or a dry vagina. Those who do not respond are a challenge, because many harsher medications have rather severe side effects, and if a patient has dry eyes and dry mouth, I do not want to give drugs that could make her feel sicker or even cause cancer.

Over the long haul, some of the very strong drugs such as cytoxan or chlorambucil, or even Imuran (azathioprine), give pause, since they have been known to increase the risk for cancer, particularly lymphoma, in patients at high risk for this disease. (We have no idea what constitutes risk, but it may be the presence of cancer-causing genes called *oncogenes* that some of us keep dormant in our cells.) I also do not believe in giving estrogen for the vaginal dryness that is caused by Sjögren's. Many gynecologists do prescribe it; seeing only the vaginal symptoms, they assume the dryness is caused by lack of hormones. As far as I am concerned, in cases of Sjögren's syndrome, and indeed in any autoimmune disease, giving estrogen is not a good idea. Estrogen actually makes the condition worse because it stimulates rather than calms the immune system.

Sometimes patients will respond only to immunosuppressive drugs to stop the cells and antibodies from attacking the glands. For those patients, I prescribe cortisone, with the dose high enough to get results but low enough not to produce the many side effects that most women abhor, including weight gain and overabundant growth of body hair.

Living with Sjögren's

Living with Sjögren's can be challenging. If the dry eyes persist despite medication, the drainage end of the tear ducts may have to be plugged surgically to keep the eyes moist. Creams and lubricants in the vagina and artificial saliva provide moisture, as mentioned above, and this seems to be sufficient for many. Patients who are very severely affected have great difficulty, however. Their eyes are chronically bloodshot and they have to wear goggles for protection. When surgery or artificial tears and saliva do not work, some patients take drugs, such as the pilocarpine preparation mentioned above, that induce as much moisture as possible, but often their mouths still are parched at times. Sjogren's patients generally require additional drugs, such as prednisone, to keep their immune systems in check and at least allow a modicum of tears and saliva. This treatment may be necessary for a lifetime. Almost all of my patients with Sjögren's are seeing psychiatrists or psychologists, not necessarily because of depression, but rather because the antibody has an effect on how their minds work. It is not an easy thing to live with this disease, but I have many patients who, despite the difficulties, continue to lead productive and enjoyable lives.

Looking to the Future

Researchers persist in their fight against Sjögren's syndrome. While searching for the cause, they are peering deeper into genetic and environmental factors that might trigger the disease. Also under investigation are treatments that will be more effective than those that are currently available, such as better ways to mimic the salivary glands and to keep dry eyes moist for longer periods of time.

The current research involves a number of very talented investigators. One large group is studying the binding of the anti-RO antibody on nerve tissue. Another is looking at the reasons that heart block appears in infants born to some mothers with Sjögren's antibodies but not all. These investigators look at newborn mice and actually study the fluorescent binding of the antibody on the heart nerves of the mouse, which also involves doing a mini-electrocardiogram on the newborn mouse. This is a remarkable operation. The probe and the machine used for this purpose are no larger than a pillbox. The idea is to find out why antibodies of a certain molecular weight affect the heart conduction system so notably, when others have no effect at all.

In another study, a group of Harvard scientists is investigating the hormones of tears and has found that the tears of patients with

Sjögren's syndrome have inadequate amounts of male hormones when compared to people without Sjögren's. This may be quite important. In other autoimmune diseases, such as lupus, we are actually contemplating the use of weakened male hormones, such as DHEA, to treat the disease. It may be helpful to do the same for patients with Sjögren's syndrome.

Laura's Story, Continued

It has been eight months since I saw Laura for the first time, and with all our therapeutic measures, she continues to do exceptionally well. With her treatment—she remains on daily prednisone to keep her immune system in check—she now is sleeping and eating normally. In addition, her saliva has returned to a great extent and she has limited tears now. She continues to use artificial tears as a supplement, though, and takes analgesics when she has joint pain. Her eyes, although often bloodshot, look well enough to allow her to return to work. The long-term conditions of chronic cough, persistently dry vagina, and so forth are taking their time to resolve, but Laura seems pleased with her progress, and to the extent that she is satisfied, so am I.

CHAPTER THIRTEEN

AUTOIMMUNE THYROID DISEASE

~~~~~

Disabling the Body's Nuclear Reactor

HE THYROID GLAND sits in the neck and is the powerhouse of the body. I like to think of it as our own personal nuclear reactor, because it controls metabolism. That is, it helps cells change chemicals into energy by secreting the necessary hormones. But the thyroid can create these hormones only if it is told to do so, and these orders come from another hormone, called thyroid-stimulating hormone (TSH). TSH is generated by the pituitary gland in the brain.

How does TSH communicate with the thyroid? If you recall, in earlier chapters I spoke of cells having receptors that lie on their surfaces. I suggested visualizing a receptor as a small lock. Because cells need to be entered if they are to receive their instructions, the lock must be opened, and that requires a specific key. In this case, the key is the hormone TSH. The communication process is as follows: TSH floating in the bloodstream recognizes the receptor for the thyroid cell. It attaches itself to the receptor and then stimulates the receptor, which in turn sends a message to the nucleus of the cell to secrete hormones. This is the normal course of events to keep the thyroid functioning as it should.

Keep this biology lesson in mind. We will return to it shortly.

The term autoimmune thyroid disease is used to describe all thyroid-related conditions caused by antibodies seeing the thyroid cells as antigens. These include the following:

▷ Graves' disease.
▷ Hashimoto's thyroiditis.
▷ Subclinical hypothyroidism (a mild elevation of TSH levels and normal circulating thyroid hormone levels).
▷ Transient thyroiditis, which includes postpartum depression.

Why the immune system attacks the thyroid is anybody's guess. When I was a student, the current belief was that certain sites of the human body were privileged, which means that for some reason, they never were exposed to the developing immune system; almost as if they were hiding in plain sight. As one gets older, however, these privileged antigens suddenly become recognized and our bodies immediately start making antigens against them.

Antibodies can beset the thyroid for a number of other reasons as well. For example, a trauma to the neck could release antigens from the thyroid itself, or infection with a virus that has a protein similar to a thyroid protein might be the culprit. Some physicians suggest that autoimmune thyroiditis may be a result of the accumulation of fetal cells in the mother's thyroid gland during pregnancy. Because Graves' disease seems to run in families, perhaps there is a genetic connection. Perhaps all of the above are true. The truth is, no one knows for sure.

Graves' disease and Hashimoto's thyroiditis are the two most prominent autoimmune thyroid diseases, accounting for approximately 90 percent of cases. Although both diseases will show antithroid antibodies in the blood, as we shall soon see, they are quite different from each other. Graves' disease causes hyperthyroidism (an overabundance of thyroid hormone) in most patients. However, depending on what is attacked by the antibody, hypothyroidism (too little hormone) in Graves' is also possible. Hashimoto's disease, in which the thyroid is either severely compromised or destroyed, is mostly responsible for too little production of hormone (hypothyroidism), but Hashimoto's can result in hyperthyroidism in rare cases. Both diseases can occur by themselves or with other autoimmune conditions, such as lupus, rheumatoid arthritis, anemia, or type 2 diabetes.

Graves' Disease

An overproduction of thyroid hormones characterizes Graves' disease. In patients with this disorder, antibodies against the thyroid-stimulating hormone receptors so closely resemble TSH that when the antibody—called *long-acting thyroid stimulator*—binds to the receptor and stimulates it, the cell thinks that the antibody is TSH and acts accordingly, by instructing the thyroid to produce thyroid hormones. Because of the thyroid's inability to differentiate between the antibody and a true stimulating hormone, the thyroid just keeps producing. This unabated stream of hormone let loose into the bloodstream is why Graves' disease is so difficult to regulate.

People with Graves' disease experience a number of symptoms, many of which are so obvious as to allow the physician to diagnose the disease merely by observing the patient. Such symptoms include:

▷ *Goiter.* This meaty mass on the neck is actually an enlarged, inflamed, and antibody-inhabited thyroid gland.
▷ *Eye protrusion.* This condition, which is known as *exopthalmos*, creates a bulging eye or staring quality to the eyes. Bulging eyes largely result from water retention, which also is accountable for the swollen tissues around the eyes.
▷ Darkening of the skin around the eyes.
▷ Weight loss despite increased appetite. This is a result of increased body metabolism.
▷ Heat intolerance.
▷ Menstrual irregularity.
▷ Mood swings.
▷ Hair loss (scalp only).

Although the disease can arise at any age, it is most frequently diagnosed for the first time in people between the ages of twenty and forty. For reasons we can only speculate about, women are affected at least twenty times more than men are. Still, plenty of men have Graves' disease. One of the best known, of course, is George Herbert Walker Bush, the forty-first president.

George H.W. Bush developed the first noticeable symptoms of this disease—shortness of breath, tightness in the chest, and a sudden feeling of overall fatigue—while golfing at Camp David on May 4, 1991. The president's physician gave him every possible test, of course, and it did not take them long to diagnose his problem as Graves' disease. In retrospect, it turned out that the president had felt tired over the preceding two weeks and had lost nine pounds over a few months, both symptoms of this condition.

It was quite fascinating to me that two years earlier, President Bush's wife, Barbara, had been diagnosed with Graves' disease, but what was truly amazing was that even their dog, Millie, had an autoimmune disease. In her case, however, it was lupus.

Treatments for Graves' disease includes drugs designed to block, or at least curtail, the runaway production of hormone. I generally prescribe *levothyroxine,* also known as L-thyroxine, for this purpose. Some people have a partial thyroidectomy or are treated with radioactive iodine, but both of these remedies, if not closely monitored, can ultimately cause hypothyroidism, or too little thyroid hormone. Untreated, patients with Graves' disease can develop fatal complications such as cardiac rhythm disturbances, muscle weakness, electrolyte imbalances, or severe constipation. Since the disease is so easy to treat, we almost never see this kind of problem.

It takes a fine balance of therapy to regulate Graves' disease, but once it is under control, the symptoms should be ameliorated. Patients are generally on therapy for the rest of their lives.

Hashimoto's Thyroiditis

Hashimoto's thyroiditis, also known as just plain thyroiditis, is *the* most common thyroid disorder. It occurs when antibodies attack the thyroid gland directly, severely affecting its function and, ultimately, leading to an insufficient production of thyroid hormone. This most common form of thyroid disease was named after Dr. Hakaru Hashimoto, who defined it in 1912.

The onset of thyroiditis is usually slow, and it may take months or even years for the condition to be detected. There may be no symptoms and no obvious physical change other than a slight gain of weight, which is common enough as we grow older. If a physician does thyroid function blood tests (TSH, T_4, and T_3), the results may even be normal at first—a negative test result—but over time they will show up intermittently as abnormal. If a patient comes to me after a negative thyroid function test, and she has no symptoms other than weight gain, I start looking for thyroid antibodies, because even if the thyroid function tests are normal, the antibody tests may be strongly positive, which would tell me that something autoimmune is going on.

Weight gain is not the only symptom to alert a physician to thyroiditis in a patient. There are many others. Notice that some of those listed below are in direct contrast to those associated with Graves' disease, but many are similar.

▷ Muscle weakness
▷ Dry or brittle hair
▷ Muscle cramps
▷ Constipation
▷ Increased risk of miscarriage
▷ Sensitivity to cold
▷ Heavy and irregular menses
▷ Difficulty concentrating or thinking
▷ Mood swings
▷ Overall fatigue

Thyroiditis strikes twenty females to every male. I have not seen a male with autoimmune thyroiditis in about fifteen years, although I see about ten cases of new thyroiditis per month in my female patients. The importance of female hormones to this clinical manifestation is apparent because of the high female preponderance, but we do not know what is the direct connection. The disease is most common in middle-aged women but can affect people in all age groups, including children. It is prevalent in people with a family history of thyroid disease. Twenty-five percent of those who have thyroiditis may develop other autoimmune diseases such as type 2 diabetes, adrenal insufficiency, or Sjögren's syndrome.

To treat thyroiditis, we try to regulate the thyroid's production of hormones and get the thyroid levels back to normal. This is best done by giving the patient lifelong thyroid hormone replacement. I usually treat the patients who have low thyroid hormone in the blood with *thyroxine*, which has many other names, such as *Synthroid*. A small pill taken once a day should be able to return the hormone in the body to normal levels. Be aware, however, that it often takes a while to determine the correct dose, and even when the dosage is correct, some women feel no better even after thyroid hormone replacement is started. Remission of hypothyroidism occurs in 5 to 10 percent of patients with Hashimoto's thyroiditis. In the others, therapy is usually lifelong.

CHAPTER FOURTEEN

AUTOIMMUNE DISEASE OF THE LIVER

~

> ## Lucky Woman Thrown by a Horse

T HE LIVER IS the body's purification factory. It is an organ full of enzymes whose primary purpose is to detoxify all the poisons that we bring to it. It cleanses us, for example, from the aspirin we ingest when the stock market drops 500 points, the one-drink-too-many on New Year's Eve, and, for many of us as we age, a whole host of drugs that make our blood pressure go down, our mood go up, our body relax, and our sexual organs rise. I have tremendous respect for this workhorse of an organ. In fact, when I am contemplating a second martini, I generally turn it down because I start seeing the image of my own *hepatocytes* (liver cells) working overtime just to keep me honest. There's always a spoiler in the house.

Generally, the liver is the purview of the gastroenterologist because it is connected to the bowel and most of the detoxification comes through our twenty-seven feet of intestine. But a specialist in my field often manages the autoimmune liver diseases, particularly *autoimmune hepatitis* and *primary biliary cirrhosis* (PBC), because in these cases it is the immune system that turns out to be the villain. Both autoimmune hepatitis and PBC are most often seen in women, and both can be life-threatening diseases.

Autoimmune Hepatitis

In autoimmune hepatitis, the immune system's T cells directly attack the liver cells, causing progressive inflammation of the liver tissue. (Hepatitis means inflammation of the liver.) This disease differs from hepatitis A, B, and C, all of which are the result of viral infections.

Autoimmune hepatitis is classified as type I and type II. There is also a newer type III autoimmune hepatitis, but no one is sure how to categorize this variant. Seventy percent of the people who get type I autoimmune hepatitis are women, most of whom range between the ages of fifteen and forty. This is the classic variety, and it is characterized by high gamma globulin levels and a variety of strange antibodies in the blood. Type II, which is not readily found in this country, generally afflicts young girls and pre-teens and is less common than type I and has antibodies specific to itself. It often is quite acute and progresses to cirrhosis in quick fashion.

In about 50 percent of patients, autoimmune hepatitis of both types exists alongside one of the other autoimmune disorders, most commonly type 1 diabetes, Hashimoto's thyroiditis, Graves' disease, or Sjögren's syndrome. This type of liver disease is extremely complex because of the unusual antigens that are derived from the cells of the liver. I strongly believe that some sort of virus, or many viruses, are responsible for this disease, but this has not yet been proven.

Left untreated, autoimmune hepatitis will most surely progress to cirrhosis, or hardening of the liver. This condition, in which scar tissue replaces normal healthy tissue, blocks the flow of blood through the organ and leaves the liver hard and fibrotic. (Alcohol-related cirrhosis is not autoimmune, of course, but the devastation of the liver is similar.) Advanced cirrhosis can lead to the liver's total destruction. Fortunately, an early diagnosis and treatment of autoimmune hepatitis can result in amelioration of the symptoms and a good prognosis, including remission.

▷ Diagnosing Autoimmune Hepatitis

Many people with autoimmune-hepatitis-related cirrhosis have no symptoms in the early stages of the disease. However, as scar tissue replaces healthy cells, liver function starts to fail and a person may experience the following:

- ▷ Exhaustion
- ▷ Fatigue
- ▷ Loss of appetite
- ▷ Weight loss
- ▷ Nausea
- ▷ Weakness

When a patient comes in to see me with suspected autoimmune liver disease, it is always after she has seen an internist or a gastroen-terologist specialist. It is likely that she went to either of those doctors with a primary complaint of fatigue and eventually developed jaundice, itching, joint pain, skin rash, or abdominal pain. The doctors could not tell her specifically what was the problem. Autoimmune hepatitis can be very difficult to diagnose, and I must admit that I, too, have missed a few cases in my day. I can order tests that seek the related antibodies, but these tests are very complex and few laboratories have them. Even if they do, the results are sensitive but not specific to the disease, meaning that the antibodies are always found in that disease, but they are found in certain other diseases as well. In addition, there can be multiple antigens at work, all of which mimic the liver cells. We do not have a clue as to what these antigens are, because autoimmune hepatitis involves so many different autoantibodies. Still, if the lab results indicate even the possibility of autoimmune hepatitis, I will follow up with a liver biopsy. This involves removing a small piece of liver tissue and examining it under a microscope to look for infiltration of immune cells in the tissue. This test can generally confirm the disease and show the extent of liver damage.

▷ *Treating Autoimmune Hepatitis*

With the diagnosis confirmed, a patient must be treated as soon as possible. The goal of treatment is to cure or at least control the disease. The best drugs we have at this point are corticosteroids, which suppress the immune system. *Imuran*, a chemotheraputic agent, also has been used with success, but it is my second choice because it can cause a form of hepatitis. Because the disease is considered more controllable than curable, even if the symptoms resolve, it may still be necessary for the patient to remain on some sort of medication long-term, if not for life. In the more advanced cases of cirrhosis, the only alternative is liver transplant, which is discussed more fully below.

Primary Biliary Cirrhosis

Primary biliary cirrhosis (PBC) is the more malignant of the autoimmune liver diseases. Whereas in autoimmune hepatitis, the antibodies are directed against the liver itself, PBC is characterized by a slow, inflammatory destruction of the small bile ducts within the liver. Bile normally leaves the liver through these ducts and ultimately drains into the intestine, where it aids in digestion. When the immune system infiltrates the bile ducts, it leaves behind inflammation and scarring that eventually clogs the ducts, resulting in severe bile backup in the liver. This condition, which is known as *bile stasis*, is highly damaging to the liver and can lead to cirrhosis and worse.

PBC is primarily a disease of women, affecting them ten times as often as men. It usually strikes between the ages of thirty and fifty-five, although older women have been known to develop the disease. Early in the disease process, patients have few, if any, symptoms—fatigue is the most common, and perhaps a subtle itching. Throughout the early stages, which can sometimes last more than a year, the only findings may be a high level of liver enzyme, called *alkaline phosphatase*, in the blood.

▷ *Trudy's Story*

I do not see many of these cases, but I am currently treating a woman named Trudy who, at the time of her first symptom, was a forty-three-year-old mother of four. Her story is quite remarkable. An avid equestrian, Trudy rode with her friends in Central Park as often as she was able, and when the children all were in school, this meant at least once a week.

For several weeks prior to her diagnosis, Trudy had not been feeling quite herself, although she could not identify what, specifically, was bothering her. She had lost some weight, although her eating habits had not changed. She had developed a subtle, if occasional, itching (*pruritus*) all over her body. When she scrutinized her skin, however, she saw no rash, no hives, no sores, or anything to explain the itch. She went to see her family doctor, who examined her, found nothing amiss, and prescribed tranquilizers, which he said were more to calm her anxiety over her itching than anything else. She told me much later that she actually never mentioned the weight loss, adding with a bit of a smile, "Why look a gift horse in the mouth?"

One Saturday morning, several weeks after she had seen her physician, her symptoms were still in evidence but so subtle as be to hardly worth mentioning again. On that morning, she went riding with a friend. The two women were cantering along the bridle path in Central Park, enjoying the beautiful summer day, when suddenly Trudy's horse bolted, throwing her into the air. She landed on the grass nearby, bruising her face and badly breaking her wrist. With the help of her friend and two nearby joggers, who hailed a taxi for her, Trudy arrived at the hospital within ten minutes of her fall.

As the orthopedist on call in the ER set Trudy's wrist, he noted a faint yellowish tinge to her skin and eyes. When he mentioned this, she told him she had not noticed, but that she'd had a few other strange symptoms. She described her itching and the weight loss. Suspecting liver disease, the doctor immediately directed her to a gastroenterologist, which she thought was strange, particularly because he stated that there was some urgency involved.

With her wrist in a cast up to her elbow, Trudy crossed to the north wing of the hospital, where a GI specialist saw her. The doctor examined her, ran some blood tests, told her she was concerned about liver disease, and promised to call her within a day or so with the results. Two days later, the call came. The doctor told Trudy she had elevated liver enzymes, and that she probably had *bile stasis* as well. This is a condition in which bile salts, unable to flow normally into the intestine, remain in the tissues. This was probably the cause of Trudy's itching. The doctor said she did not know what was the cause of the elevated enzymes, but could rule out hepatitis because Trudy's liver was not enlarged or tender, which is always found with hepatitis. Also, her hepatitis blood test was negative, but other blood tests showed that Trudy was positive for antimitochondria and anti-smooth muscle antibodies, the two most prominent antibodies that are associated with PBC.

Ultimately, Trudy received a preliminary diagnosis of PBC, and her gastroenterologist referred her to me. When I saw Trudy, she was still only mildly jaundiced, but from her tests it was clear that something was brewing in her liver. I felt I needed a liver biopsy to define precisely what it was. I tried to explain to her the possible seriousness of her condition, but she had a hard time believing it because she felt so well. I explained that many people with PBC have no symptoms in the early stages of the disease, but as scar tissue replaces healthy cells, liver function starts to fail and the symptoms become more noticeable.

I sent Trudy for a biopsy the next day. Sometimes I will first order an ultrasound or a radioisotope liver scan, but I had the feeling time was going to be of the essence in this case, and it turned out I was correct. The biopsy showed a considerable amount of bile in her tissues, meaning that her bile ducts were congested to the point of overflowing. Trudy indeed had bile stasis. The biopsy also showed that her disease had progressed to the point at which her liver was hardened and shrinking in size—two classic symptoms of primary biliary cirrhosis. Trudy was clearly in growing danger. If the disease progressed much further, no matter how well she felt, her liver could shut down altogether.

I admitted her to the hospital immediately. I put her on intravenous cortisone and other immunosuppressive drugs to try to slow the rapidly dividing immune cells, but neither of these drugs seemed to alter the course of the disease. I then switched her to *ursodeoxycholic acid*, a pill that helps alleviate the symptoms of the bile backup, relieves the itching, and dissolves any gallstones that may occur. This fairly new drug can make liver tissue come alive, but it is not perfect because at a certain point it loses its effects. In Trudy, even this drug did not stop the progression as effectively as I had hoped. As the antibodies continued their assault on her liver, I could see that it was just a matter of time before she would require a liver transplant. We put her name on the national registry, and she went home to wait.

Liver transplantation is now an accepted form of treatment for advanced chronic liver disease. The success rate improves daily, and survival rates at transplant centers are now well over 90 percent, with excellent quality of life after recovery. The problem, as with all organs, is the scarcity of livers. Within a number of weeks, Trudy was fortunate enough to receive an excellent match from someone who refused to wear a helmet and ultimately crashed his motorcycle. She did extremely well and today, a year later, she is leading a normal life and riding her horse again. Interestingly, it is rare for a transplated liver to become cirrhotic. No one quite knows why that is, but we are not complaining.

Trudy is lucky, and she knows it. If you ask her why, she'll tell you it is because her horse threw her. She says she often wonders what would have happened had her horse been looking left instead of right. In that case, he might not have seen the obstacle that caused him to bolt and Trudy to fall. Had she continued her ride that glorious day, would she have known of the destruction that was silently assaulting her liver? Maybe yes, maybe no. Maybe yes, but too late. Had she not broken her arm, which brought her to the hospital where she met the orthopedist who waved the red flag that eventually got her the treatment she required, she might not have been so fortunate.

CHAPTER FIFTEEN

SCLERODERMA

❦

The Woman with Thick Skin

"LET'S GO BACK around fourteen months," Dee said.

Dee is a children's book editor. She is warm and sensitive with sparkling blue eyes and an amazing love of life. But on the day we met, the way she got right to things and the straightforward manner in which she spoke gave me the feeling she had sat across from numerous physicians before me and recited this litany many times—too many to suit her. "Imagine this: You're thirty-one years old. You're in a new city. You've got a new job. You're on a blind date in a fabulous restaurant with a man who, it just so happens, turns out to be more handsome than you could ever have hoped. You're talking and you're eating and you're not believing your luck when suddenly, *bam*! Out of the blue you begin to choke."

I shook my head at the visual image, and she continued.

"I felt like there was food stuck in my throat and I couldn't get it up. Amazingly, some man at the next table rushed over and did the Heimlich maneuver, but nothing emerged. Then, suddenly, I was okay. Can you imagine how mortifying that is, on a first date? It was awful. Fortunately, when it was over, we decided to forget the whole incident and got on with the evening."

Dee stood up and paced around the room, helped herself to some water, and continued. "For the next four days I was left with a feeling of dull ache in my chest area, almost in the same spot where I felt the food stick. I was petrified to eat anything other than soft food for a while, but eventually I began to eat normally again. Then, one afternoon I was eating a hamburger and it happened again, except now I knew I wasn't choking. Right around then, too, I began experiencing these periodic waves of fatigue. I figured they were because I was working hard during the day and staying out late with Jeff at night. Eventually, though, it became a tremendous effort to stay awake past nine. Not the greatest thing when you've just started a relationship."

Dee, who had only a few years ago been a member of the track team at Florida State University, went on to tell me that she was now sleeping almost eleven hours per night and, upon awakening, still did not feel refreshed. The next symptoms developed perhaps a few weeks later, a shortness of breath, a slight but persistent cough, and a drop in her weight, which was not that welcome because she has a lean runner's body to begin with. She went to a new internist, who did a workup that included a battery of blood tests, and everything came back normal. He dutifully suggested that she rest when she was tired, take vitamins, eat solid meals, and drink a milkshake daily until she put back the weight she had recently lost. She complied with every one of his suggestions, and two months later, when things did not get better, she added depression to her list of symptoms.

"It was the unbearable, overwhelming exhaustion, that was getting me down more than anything," she told me, a look of sheer frustration on her face. "And no one could find anything to hang a diagnosis on." At the suggestion of one physician, she reluctantly went to see a psychiatrist. To his credit, when she described her unremitting shortness of breath, dry cough, and lack of energy he sent her directly to a lung specialist. After a series of tests, the pulmonologist asked Dee if she felt any tightness in her hands. Thinking this a strange question, she told him that she had, and not in the joints but more in the skin, and this only very recently. The physician told Dee that she did indeed have what he called "a real condition," and that she should make an appointment with a rheumatologist.

From the time she felt her first symptom in the restaurant to the time she finally came to see me, seventeen months had passed. Unfortunately, this is not an unusual amount of time when it comes to diagnosing as elusive a disease as *scleroderma*. When I told Dee I felt this might be what she had, like so many of my patients, she expressed tremendous relief that she had, as she called it, "something."

One of the hardest parts of working in this field is seeing patients at the end of an exhaustive, frustrating journey toward a diagnosis. I wish there was a way to cut through all the superfluous doctors' visits along the path, but there does not seem to be. Not yet, anyway. And I understand how it can happen. Because she was a new patient, Dee's internist did not know her well enough to be able to diagnose what he could not see, feel, or measure. Tiredness and weight loss are common complaints in a variety of diseases of both the mind and the body, and the symptoms are so subjective that they can elicit different responses from different physicians. That is why it is so important that patients and physicians get to know each other, no easy task given the few short minutes allotted to each visit. In any case, had he known her better, Dee's doctor could have determined immediately that she was not malingering. To the contrary, she is a high-energy woman in every sense of the word. But until there are definitive tests for these esoteric diseases, or until every doctor in America is educated to look for them, I have a feeling for many years to come, patients like Dee will be sitting across my desk, emitting a similar sigh of relief.

In any case, now that Dee had a diagnosis, her plight had only just begun.

What Is Scleroderma?

Scleroderma, which is also known as *progressive systemic sclerosis*, literally means "hard skin." It is a chronic autoimmune disease that affects the blood vessels and the connective tissue—the tendons, muscles, joints, and organ coverings. First discovered in the eighteenth century, today scleroderma afflicts up to 50,000 Americans, primarily women between the ages of thirty and fifty at onset. Women are up to five times more likely than men to get this disease. The degree of scleroderma varies from patient to patient; it can be a nuisance to some and life-threatening to others. There is no cure.

There are two main types of scleroderma: localized and systemic:

Localized scleroderma. More common in children, localized scleroderma is divided into two categories: morphea and linear scleroderma. In both cases, localized scleroderma affects a specific area of the skin but not the internal organs. Morphea refers to one or more small patches of thick, tight skin that can occur anywhere on the body. Morphea usually develops over a period of years, then fades, and the skin texture returns to normal, although there may be some pigment changes. Linear describes the same type of patches when they develop in a line down one arm or leg or on the face.

Systemic scleroderma. Often called *internal* scleroderma, it is more common in adults, and affects the skin, internal organs, and gastrointestinal tract (see symptoms later). It can also affect the musculoskeletal system. There are two classifications of systemic scleroderma: limited and diffuse. Limited scleroderma tends to result in less severe organ problems than diffuse. Diffuse scleroderma comes on faster than limited and exhibits many different patterns, as we will see. Dee has diffuse systemic scleroderma.

One of the most famous people, certainly the most famous artist, to develop scleroderma was Paul Klee, a German citizen who was born in Switzerland in 1879. Klee was a teacher and a pioneer in modern art. He developed the disease in 1935 at the age of fifty-six. For a year before that, he had lived with unrelenting fatigue. As there were no definitive tests for scleroderma then (there are still none), the fatigue was thought to be associated with a severe case of measles he had recently experienced. After a while, however, on noticing a subtle change in his skin, his doctors began to suspect scleroderma. Shortly thereafter, photographs of Klee's hands were taken and compared with photographs of his hands taken a decade earlier. The newly taut skin was remarkably noticeable and provided verification of the diagnosis. His prodigious artistic talent, even after his diagnosis became known (and at a time when there were very few drugs to treat the symptoms of scleroderma), became an example of the spirit of people who have scleroderma and yet continue to function as though nothing is different. I keep a small watercolor of Paul Klee's on my desk at home to remind me of his indomitable character and the resilience of the human spirit.

What Causes Scleroderma?

In patients with scleroderma, it is believed that the immune system is attacking the connective tissue, although in truth, no one knows for sure what the target is. We do know that the attack leaves behind scar tissue, or fibrosis, which leads to degenerative changes in the skin, blood vessels, and skeletal muscle. Internal organs are affected, too, including the heart, kidneys, and gastrointestinal tract, part of which is the esophagus, as we saw with Dee. As the disease progresses, scar tissue builds up and causes the normally soft tissue to harden. As an illustrative example, consider a scab that appears on the skin after a wound. If you have ever tried to bend a scab, you have an idea how tough the material is. This is the same fibrotic material that builds up within the skin or organs of the body of a person with scleroderma.

What triggers this particular disease remains a mystery. Some of the possibilities include having a genetic predisposition to it, contracting a virus, or being exposed to certain chemicals. We do not understand much about the genetic aspect of scleroderma other than to say there may be a gene that makes one susceptible to the factors that trigger the disease. In other words, a person must have a specific genetic makeup as well as a particular trigger to be vulnerable to scleroderma. The trigger might be a rogue virus or some chemical or toxic substance in the environment.

Some eighteen years ago, there was an epidemic in Spain in which some 20,000 people became ill from rapeseed oil, a toxic substance that looks and tastes like olive oil and had been substituted illegally for it in that country. People who ingested this oil became profoundly disfigured and disabled with what came to be called toxic oil syndrome. I saw slides of the victims at a medical meeting and can still recall the photographs of their faces, which had stiff foreheads, hyperpigmented skin, and tight purse-string mouths. No one at the meeting could distinguish the physical symptoms of scleroderma from those caused by the toxic oil, that's how closely they resembled each other.

Although there appears to be no direct connection between sclero-derma and toxic oil syndrome, the possibility looms large that sclero-derma is an environmentally caused disease. Many people who are exposed to certain chemicals such as arsenic, vinyl chloride, or even coal dust have been known to develop scleroderma. Sadly, some pa-tients undergoing chemotherapy for cancer acquire scleroderma from chemotheraputic drugs such as *bleomycin.*

One possible cause of scleroderma that has been of great interest to scientists and physicians alike is the chimeric cell. As I mentioned in chapter 2, a chimeric cell is one that floats in the body of one person yet has the HLA, that is, the inherited genes, of someone else. There are only a few ways such a cell can enter a body. Generally, the ex-change takes place during pregnancy or delivery. For example, we know that during the period of gestation, a fetus's cells contain both the mother's and the father's HLA types. It is possible that while in the uterus, a mother's placental circulation might come into contact with her child's as he or she floats in the cushioned amniotic fluid. In other words, the fetus might bleed a few cells into the mother's circu-lation, or the mother's cells might be transferred to the baby. Such a cell (or cells) can remain in the body for years, even decades. These cells do not divide like normal cells, they just continue to circulate around in the bloodstream, inducing a heightened responsiveness in the mother's immune system. In other words, the body knows some-thing may be amiss, but is not sure what. Then, one day, for no ap-parent reason, the stranger cell is suddenly right there in the open, for the immune system to see. When that occurs, the immune response results, the T cells go on the attack, and the response that results is called a graft-versus-host (GVH) disease. This is thought to precipi-tate the disease scleroderma. (It can also precipitate other illnesses, such as lupus.)

Symptoms of Scleroderma

Listed below are some of the classic symptoms for scleroderma. While Dee had a number of them, she escaped others, which also is typical of this disease. It is so unpredictable that you can never say with any assurance who will get which symptoms or when. Nor can you say in whom the disease will progress and in whom it will plateau. These are topics for researchers in the future, if they are not already being studied.

▷ *Sclerodactyly of the Skin*

The most well known symptom of scleroderma is *sclerodactyly*, in which the skin becomes smooth, shiny, and tight with a loss of subcutaneous tissue. Not everyone who has scleroderma gets sclerosis of the skin, but those who do can experience symptoms across the body in small or large areas, including the chest, the torso, the back, and the upper and lower legs. When sclerosis occurs over the fingers, as it generally does first, they may not be as flexible as they normally were. Small, painful ulcers may appear on the tips of the fingers, which can be accompanied by changes in pigment. (Skin can be hypo- or hyperpigmented, that is, the color can become lighter or darker, on various parts of the body.) When skin over the face tightens, facial expression becomes difficult and the opening of the mouth becomes restricted, producing an expression often referred to as "purse-string mouth" because of the contracted nature of the lips. This symptom can and often does occur along with the symptoms of internal scleroderma.

▷ *Fatigue*

Symptoms of extreme fatigue are common to most of the illnesses in this book and add a layer of trouble to the process of diagnosing almost every one of them. Fatigue can be mild, in which case just a short nap can ease the symptom, or it can be unrelenting and overwhelming, superseding all daily activity. My patients tell me that the devastation that comes with autoimmune-related fatigue is indescribable. It is the one symptom most of them complain of first, and certainly it is almost always mentioned by women with scleroderma.

▷ *Raynaud's Phenomenon*

Maurice Raynaud, a French doctor, characterized this very common herald of scleroderma first at the time of the Civil War. Doctor Raynaud described a condition in which the fingertips become so sensitive to cold that the capillaries nearest the skin shut down, a process known as vasoconstriction. When this happens, color changes occur in the fingers and toes, starting from red (good blood flow) to blue (blood slows and eventually stops), to white (total lack of blood flow.) I have actually heard this called a "patriotic disease." When the fingers or toes turn white, they begin to sting, and after a few minutes they can become numb.

Raynaud's can affect one or two fingers on one or both hands, symptoms vary from person to person, and the blanching and pain never last longer than thirty minutes. This phenomenon can also occur in the toes, the nose, and even the ears.

In patients with severe scleroderma, Raynaud's symptoms occur more often, and the chronic interruption of blood flow to a finger can ultimately result in painful ulcers at the tip. Furthermore, because of lack of oxygen at the tip, the finger pads may lose fat and become pointy (diagnostically referred to as penciling), skin may die, and eventually portions or all of the digit, including some bone, may be lost. Some people do not know that they have Raynaud's until they realize there is a sore on a fingertip that refuses to heal. That is when they generally go to their doctor.

In Dee's case, Raynaud's symptoms appeared a year before her other symptoms, but she did not know what it meant, nor did she consider it to be anything more than an annoyance. She was smart enough to wear gloves when it was cold, which most people will do, and as so much of her time was spent in Florida, she had symptoms only when she went into strongly air conditioned rooms and not always then.

I should note that Raynaud's is referred to as Raynaud's *phenomenon* when it appears with another disease, such as scleroderma, and Raynaud's disease when it stands alone. Many women can have Raynaud's disease all of their lives, and it may never be associated with scleroderma or any other disease for that matter. Raynaud's can be treated in several ways. I prefer the simple technique of swinging the arm around like a Ferris wheel, which promotes centrifugal force. By its very nature, it forces the blood vessels to dilate, and sends blood to the fingertips. In some cases, I will prescribe medication such as procardia or diltiazem, which relaxes the blood vessels, allowing flow to the tips of the extremities.

▷ *Hypertension and Kidney Disease*

A potentially serious symptom of scleroderma transpires when collagen builds up on the inner walls of the blood vessels and restricts the flow of blood through the vessel. The diminished flow of blood creates a lack of pressure to many areas in the body, including the renal arteries to the kidney. When the kidneys sense a low arterial pressure, they are fooled into believing they need to raise certain blood chemicals to keep the flow of blood constant in the rest of the body. The result is severe hypertension and kidney disease. If the pressure becomes high enough, it can cause a stroke, which, at its very worst, can be fatal.

▷ *Swallowing Difficulty*

As we saw with Dee, scleroderma often results in dysfunction at the lower end of the esophagus, leading to a tightening of the muscle at the esophageal sphincter, where the esophagus joins the stomach. This can sometimes result in spasm of the esophagus upon swallowing and in blockage of food entering the stomach, both of which can manifest themselves as chest pain. (Doctors see any number of patients each year who believe that they are having a heart attack when in fact they are having esophageal spasm.) Sometimes this symptom manifests itself in a feeling of fullness at the stomach area. If the swallowing becomes too difficult or the feeling of fullness extremely uncomfortable, patients stop eating solid foods. When the bowel is affected, it becomes stiff with collagen, and the absorption of food diminishes, leading to severe diarrhea and weight loss.

▷ *Reflux*

A second gastrointestinal symptom, also associated with swallowing problems, is gastroesophageal reflux disease (GERD). In this case, the esophageal sphincter does not close properly and allows stomach acid to back up into the esophagus. The sensation is one of burning belching. This is no small case of heartburn—it really hurts! Stress makes it worse because it increases acid in the stomach. So does ingesting caffeine, alcohol, and other highly acidic foods.

▷ *Shortness of Breath*

One of the most perplexing symptoms of this and many other autoimmune diseases is *pulmonary fibrosis*—a thickening of the tissue of the lungs, which compromises lung function and prevents patients from getting enough oxygen. When Dee's lung specialist looked at her chest X-ray, he saw normal lungs, but when he had her breathe into a machine that assesses pulmonary function and then looked at the exchange of oxygen and carbon dioxide, he saw the problem. Pulmonary fibrosis, scar tissue buildup in the lungs, hindered the exchange of oxygen and carbon dioxide and accounted for much of Dee's shortness of breath and certainly her overall feelings of tiredness. She simply could not get enough oxygen into her lungs, particularly at times of exertion when she needed it most. When Dee was given oxygen to breathe, she became more comfortable. She also learned not to inhale too deeply because when she did, she began to cough.

Diagnosing Scleroderma

It would be effortless to diagnose scleroderma if the symptoms were in evidence from day one, but this is not the nature of the beast, at least not this beast. When Dee was initially examined, the findings were not obvious. Her physicians were technically accurate in their diagnoses, based on what they saw, particularly since few physicians, especially specialists in other fields, see more than one or two cases of scleroderma, if that, in a career. I have seen patients who have gone years before achieving a diagnosis of an autoimmune disease simply because fatigue and weakness were the overriding symptoms.

With scleroderma, it is essential to determine the extent of internal involvement and to do studies that provide a baseline for future evaluations. I wanted to get Dee through the tests as quickly as possible because she had already lost so much time.

▷ *Laboratory Workup*

Blood tests are not very useful for diagnosing scleroderma except to help define whether the disease is flying solo or is part of another condition. The only blood test I consider beneficial is one that isolates the scleroderma antibody, called the SCL 70 or *antitopoisomerase*. This antibody is not the cause of scleroderma, as far as we currently know, but if it appears in the blood, that is very suggestive of scleroderma, meaning that the disease *may* exist. Only about 25 percent of patients with scleroderma have this antibody, however, which is why it is considered suggestive *of*, not specific *to*, the disease. Personally, I find very few positive cases of scleroderma by way of blood evaluation, which is why I much prefer to make the diagnosis the old-fashioned way: by listening to and examining my patient.

▷ X-rays

Because of her difficulty in swallowing, I arranged first for Dee to have a "barium swallow," for which she prepared by eating a barium-laced hamburger. Barium is a heavy element that is opaque on X-ray. Combining it with a particular food allows me to actually watch that food progress down the esophagus and into the stomach. I also ordered a barium study of her small bowel to confirm the presence of a configuration of bowel loops specific to scleroderma. Barium studies are not done as often today as they were several years ago. The current gold standard test for most gastrointestinal illnesses is an endoscopy (i.e., colonoscopy and esophagogastroscopy). But for patients with scleroderma, the barium series, although not always pleasant for the patient, is still useful for identifying a change in the bowel-wall patterns.

As it turned out, the X-ray showed that the motility of Dee's esophagus muscles was poor and she had the classic "bird-beak" sign, in which the esophagus looks narrowed at the base, like a bird beak. The narrowing allows food to accumulate and ultimately leads to a sense of fullness, indigestion, severe discomfort, and pain. I also was able to evaluate the muscle tone of the sphincter at the juncture where the esophagus meets the stomach.

With her diagnosis assured, our next step was to lay out a treatment plan.

Treating Scleroderma

I wish I could say differently, but as with most other autoimmune diseases, we cannot cure the underlying process in this illness. The good news, though, is that the survival of patients with scleroderma has increased dramatically over the past ten years. This improvement reflects our ability to diagnose the disease earlier and to treat the life-threatening conditions, such as kidney disease.

Because scleroderma affects so many different parts of the body, and because there are several different classifications of this disease, there can be no universal treatment plan that works for everyone. But of late, we have been quite successful in treating many of the symptoms. For example, there are now drugs to lower high blood pressure, ease swallowing difficulties, and even increase breathing capacity. Reflux is quite manageable by lifestyle modification—giving up smoking and avoiding foods such as those containing caffeine, tomatoes, and alcohol, which can increase stomach acid. I also suggest medication for reflux.

A number of very new and, in some cases, still experimental drugs for scleroderma are currently in trials. Some of these have performed to a minor degree, but as you will see, more have had very disappointing results. I think they all bear mentioning anyway because certain uses of these drugs may, in time, prove effective. I have on more than one occasion seen a drug fail in its initial purpose, only to serendipitously become a godsend for another illness. Here are some of them:

▷ *Thalidomide.* This drug of the 1960s, associated with birth defects, is currently under investigation as a therapy for scleroderma because it is a marvelous immunosuppressant. The drug was originally released as a tranquilizer. Today, its only bad side effects are the numbness and tingling that occurs in the arms and the legs, which in most cases is irreversible. To date, the results of using this drug for scleroderma have been disappointing. *Warning: Pregnant women should never take thalidomide for any reason.*

▷ *Anti-TGF.* One of the most recent experimental treatments is a yet-unnamed drug designed to block tissue growth factor

(TGF). TGF is a cytokine that we think plays a role in the laying down of fibrous tissue. If TGF can be blocked, it might arrest the scar tissue buildup that makes this disease so potentially devastating.

▷ *Para-amino benzoic acid (PABA)*. Used in sunscreen, PABA is known to soften skin to varying degrees. Used topically, however, it will not affect the internal organs. Practically speaking, it would be more efficacious to take PABA by mouth, and it does come in pill form, but the pill is large and must be taken in large numbers (as many as twenty per day), which presents a problem for people who cannot swallow well.

▷ *Penicillamine*. Not related to the more common penicillin, penicillamine has been used for years to treat scleroderma. Penicillamine can soften the skin for some people, but most people have little success with the drug.

▷ *Relaxin*. A natural hormone that helps the uterus relax during childbirth. It was hoped that relaxin could be synthesized and used to soften skin or relax esophageal stiffening to avoid the problems associated with swallowing, but the results of early studies employing it have not been promising.

Pregnancy and Scleroderma

Women who have scleroderma can become pregnant but if I am asked, I tend to advise against it. It is very difficult for scleroderma patients to become pregnant, and delivering the baby is not only tough but can be extremely complicated, particularly if the disease is of an internal nature.

Living with Scleroderma: Dee's Story

Dee has done remarkably well with drugs that treat her symptoms. She is taking *metoclopramide* to relax the muscle in the base of her esophagus, so swallowing has become much easier and she no longer experiences the sensation of food being caught in her throat. For her GERD, she takes a proton pump inhibitor (Nexium) to decrease the amounts of acid in her stomach and to prevent her GERD from keeping her awake at night. Blood flow to her fingers has been restored with a class of drugs called *calcium channel blockers*. These drugs act as vasodilators, relaxing the blood vessels and making it easier for blood to flow through. Relaxed blood vessels mean less pressure against the vessel walls, which lowers the blood pressure, so she has a double benefit.

Living with scleroderma has not been easy. The skin on her hands is tightening to the degree that two of her fingers have become gnarled and she is having trouble bending a few of the others. The pigment on her hands is changing and turning darker. On some days, she finds it hard to eat without drinking a great deal of fluid to help the food travel down her esophagus. Dee's most debilitating symptom, fatigue, cannot as yet be treated effectively, but she and her husband Jeff—yes, she married the guy—have learned to make it part of their day and treat it accordingly.

Hope springs eternal in this illness. Dee says she is determined to lead a fairly normal life, and that she is prepared to face the many annoyances that attend her condition. She has given up alcohol and placed the head of her bed up on three-inch blocks to decrease her gastric irritation, and she puts hydrating cream such as Lubriderm or Aveeno Oil on her body daily to keep her skin soft. Of course, she has some complaints, but they are usually about small, bothersome things, such as the fact that she cannot play a guitar, which, as she readily admits, may be a blessing to those listening. Still, she manages quite well within her limitations. She continues to edit books, to travel with Jeff, and to do the things she loves. Each time I see her, she says that she can only hope that one day we will be able to make her soft again. I certainly hope so, too.

CHAPTER SIXTEEN

POLYMYOSITIS AND DERMATOMYOSITIS

Ragged Fibers

*I*T IS NO secret that physicians sometimes label their patients. No, I don't mean we refer to them as "the appendix in room 312 by the door," as I admit I sometimes did in medical school. Rather, I mean we often speak of these patients with great *pride*. "I'm treating a best-selling author," one physician might say while sitting at a breakfast meeting with his colleagues. "Oh," another might interject, "I just diagnosed 'X,' the conductor of our local symphony." Well, in that vein I suppose I would just jump right in and brag about Victoria, my "ballerina."

Vicki is not a professional. Far from it. Rather, she is a woman in her late thirties who is madly and passionately in love with this particular dance form, doing it, that is, not watching it. She looks the part, too. She is slender and leggy and every time I see her, her hair is pulled back tightly into a ballerina's knot. By her own admission, before her illness struck, her job as a marketing manager for a small startup computer company was merely a means to pay for ballet classes. "It's an out-of-control passion, I admit it," she told me at our first meeting. She had arrived at that meeting moving very slowly and tenuously, in much the same way as my rheumatoid arthritis (RA) patients describe their early morning hours. I could see the frustration in her face.

We spoke for a while, and I learned of her passion for ballet. When I asked why she had never become a professional dancer, she told me she was too tall. "I'm five foot, nine inches tall and *en pointe*, I'm over six feet. In ballet, that just doesn't cut it, unfortunately. But still, no one could possibly love it more than I do." Then followed the plea I was expecting: "Which is why you have to help me, Doctor Lahita. Not dancing is simply not an option."

Vicki explained that she noticed her first symptoms while taking a dance class. "We were warming up before class and I tried to raise my leg to get my heel on the barre for a stretch. But I couldn't do it. My leg just wouldn't lift! That had never happened before. Thinking it was just a bad day or that I was tired, I just put a lot of effort into it and went on with the class. I forgot about it, until two days later in another class. When I went into a plie, I couldn't get back up again. My thigh muscles refused to respond. I figured I must have the flu, so I left class early and vowed to take the next week off, which I did. The following Monday, on my way to work, I could hardly muster the strength to climb the two flights up from the subway, and that was when I knew something had to be wrong."

As Vicki's symptoms worsened, she began to make the rounds of doctors. Before coming to me, she had been to her internist, a chiropractor, an acupuncturist, and an orthopedist. It was the orthopedist who suggested that she might have an autoimmune disease, and he referred her to me. After reading the reports she brought with her and doing a cursory examination, and after taking into consideration her otherwise good health, her gender, and her age, I immediately suspected that she had an autoimmune muscle disease, of which there are two: *polymyositis* and *dermatomyositis*.

The Muscle Diseases: An Overview

Polymyositis (PM) and dermatomyositis (DM) provoke symptoms leading to muscle weakness and subsequent muscle atrophy. These *inflammatory myopathies*—as they are sometimes known—are characterized by swollen, degenerative, and symmetrical changes in the muscles (*polymyositis*) and often in the skin as well as muscle (*dermatomyositis*). While DM is distinguished from PM by the addition of a characteristic rash, the muscle inflammation and other symptoms are similar.

Polymyositis generally affects people above age twenty; dermatomyositis is seen in adults but is also found in children starting around age five. Both conditions can and often do overlap with other autoimmune diseases, including lupus, vasculitis, and Sjögren's syndrome. Thyroid diseases such as Hashimoto's thyroiditis or Graves' disease (see chapter 13) also may affect the muscles in ways similar to the inflammatory myositides, but they generally cause weakness without the associated muscle damage. Raynaud's phenomenon (see pages 174–175) also has been linked to these two diseases.

Muscle is an easy target for the immune system, if only because of its size. Our bodies are 40 percent muscle. Muscles come in three varieties: *smooth, cardiac,* and *striated.* Smooth muscle is made of fibers in uniform lengths and operates within the bowels and blood vessels, rectum, bladder, and uterus. It is even present in the pupils of our eyes. Cardiac muscle is well known to us all as that irreplaceable—well, almost irreplaceable—mass that silently pulsates within us, beating seventy or so times a minute in my chest as I sit writing this, and in yours as you are reading it. (And 800 times in the hummingbird just outside my window.)

Despite our reverence for the heart muscle, it is the striated muscle (one fiber bridges across to the next) to which we pay the most attention in our daily lives. The striated muscle helps us win a tennis match from a rival, change a blown-out tire, and lift a sleeping baby. It is the striated muscle that hurts when we run marathons and gets flabby when we ignore it completely. When the autoantibody goes hunting, it is the striated muscle, for some unknown reason, on which it sets its crosshairs.

What causes an antibody to see muscle tissue as an antigen? Nobody knows, but we think that unknown viruses may play a role. These viruses probably infect the muscle cells, causing them to express antigens on their surface, which then makes them appear foreign to the immune system. Not everyone will be susceptible to the virus, however. You have to be genetically predisposed in order to be affected by it. In other words, let's say a virus has been set loose to circulate in a small room full of people. Some people will get devastatingly ill from that virus, and others will just fend it off like a cold. Some are susceptible, others are not. No one knows why.

I should mention, too, that polymyositis and dermatomyositis have been anecdotally reported in some women with silicone breast implants, but the significance of this association has not been proven. (See chapter 18 for more on this topic.)

There are many other myositic diseases that are not autoimmune but bear mentioning. HIV and Coxsackie virus can induce syndromes similar to polymyositis. The drug penicillamine and, recently, a variety of newer drugs called *statins*, which are used to lower cholesterol, have been found to cause muscle inflammation and weakness—symptoms that can look exactly like the autoimmune forms of the disease. Myositis has also followed Botox injections, but whether there is an autoimmune relationship is unknown. I have my doubts. Still, if you are wondering if this is a reason not to get Botox injections, my very unscientific response is: It is probably a roll of the dice.

Polymyositis

When polymyositis-associated muscle weakness occurs, it generally begins in the limbs, particularly in those segments of the limbs closest to the trunk. (In medicine, the region closest to the center of the body is called the *proximal* area, and the one farthest is known as the *distal* area.) Advanced cases of the disease can eventually spread beyond the knees and elbows and to the hands and feet and other regions of the body. Polymyositis develops slowly over a period of time and often goes unnoticed until it starts to affect everyday life, as it happened with Vicki. In addition to muscle weakness, patients may have fatigue and intermittent fever and may have difficulty sitting and standing from a seated position. Patients also complain of difficulty sleeping, chewing, swallowing, and even breathing.

Dermatomyositis

Dermatomyositis is similar to polymyositis but is characterized in addition by a rash that usually comes on before the muscle weakness. This patchy, dusky purplish rash may appear on the face, shoulders, neck, trunk, elbows, or knees. There may also be small, violet-colored nodules on the knuckles and purple rashes around the eyes, suggestive of raccoon's eyes. This disease often causes joint pain in addition to muscle weakness and may be associated with a gastrointestinal malignancy. No one knows why there is an association with malignancy or cancer, but it may result from a substance excreted by the tumor that floats around the body, eventually encountering and altering the muscle cells. The altered muscle cells then look foreign to the patient's immune system, which ultimately attacks the muscles. It is important to understand that *dermatomyositis is not cancer; it is a by-product of cancer.* Accordingly, if a woman (or man) is in her fifties or sixties when she develops dermatomyositis, doctors know to immediately look for a tumor, particularly if the disease arises suddenly.

Diagnosing the Inflammatory Myopathies

It is not as difficult to diagnose the inflammatory myopathies as it is most other autoimmune diseases because the symptoms are so obvious, particularly to the rheumatologist. The diminishing muscle strength is a fair giveaway for those with polymyositis, and the distinctive dermatomyositis rash is unmistakable. Still, it is essential to take every step possible to make sure the diagnosis is accurate. This includes the following, not necessarily in order:

▷ *Complete patient history.* While the history alone may provide clues as to whether a patient has definite muscle weakness or merely muscle fatigue, it also provides a baseline for subsequent evaluations.
▷ *Physical examination.* The physician must examine the patient thoroughly to determine the strength of the muscles and to establish the presence of and severity of any weakness.

▷ *Enzyme tests.* Autoimmune-related muscle diseases release specific muscle enzymes into the circulation, particularly *creatine kinase* (CK), the enzyme tested for most often because of its sensitivity and specificity to striated muscle, or another enzyme called *aldolase*. Enzyme tests are all done using a patient's blood sample. An elevated CK or aldolase can accompany or predict this autoimmune disease. Even in older cases, in which the symptoms have resolved or stabilized after treatment, an elevated CK or aldolase can warn of an impending relapse. CK or aldolase levels are not always the last word in diagnosis, however, because people with no disease can experience elevated levels of both enzymes, and occasionally a person may have active disease and no elevated enzyme levels.

▷ *Additional blood tests.* Other tests are given to look for certain autoantibodies in the blood. Antinuclear and anticytoplasmic antibodies are common in polymyositis and dermatomyositis, but they are not specific. Finding them in the blood does not necessarily mean the disease exists. It is one more *clue* pointing in the right direction, however. Finding *synthetase* antibodies in the blood—those related to the building of new muscles—also can be helpful in making the diagnosis, but these antibodies are generally very hard to measure.

▷ *Electromyography (EMG).* This test involves placing tiny needles within the muscle and sending a series of electrical stimuli though the needles to see how the muscle responds. The typical waves of the person with polymyositis are erratic and of low amplitude. Although this test can help to provide an accurate diagnosis, it goes against my grain as a physician, reminding me of the day I took the Hippocratic oath and pledged to "do no harm." In short, an EMG hurts, and I hate to do it. But I do, because it is useful in documenting muscle weakness and in differentiating myopathies from neuropathy.

▷ *Muscle biopsy.* Perhaps the most conclusive test for polymyositis and dermatomyositis, this procedure involves removing a tiny segment of muscle with a small needle. Structural changes in the muscles of someone with this disease vary greatly, and include degeneration and even death of muscle fibers. In cases of dermatomyositis, the biopsy evaluates at the skin to determine the presence and extent of atrophy and lymphocyte infiltration.

▷ *Muscle imaging/ultrasound.* Occasionally, if an EMG or muscle biopsy is normal and particular antibodies are not present, an ultrasound may be helpful because it can show inflammation as well as atrophy of the muscle.

When I looked under the microscope at the tissue samples from some of Vicki's affected muscles, I was astonished to see such a preponderance of lymphocytes. Millions of white cells were infiltrating the muscles themselves and causing massive muscle destruction. She was still mobile, if very weak and uncomfortable, but I knew that she would not be able to continue for long, however, because her affected muscles were losing ground fast. They were actually being liquefied by the attack of the lymphocytes.

Knowing that treatment with certain drugs could stop the total destruction of her muscles, I admitted Vicki to the hospital immediately. I gave her a *bolus* (high initial dose) of intravenous prednisone in an effort to slow down (if not stop) her immune reaction, free her from pain, and get her moving again. Prednisone, Imuran, and cytoxan generally work well for this purpose. Unfortunately, they did not work for Vicki. Despite the high dosage, she did not improve. In fact, her muscles became painful even to the lightest touch. I should mention here that even if it had worked, I probably would not have kept her on steroids for very long because of the side effects. The use of corticosteroids always must be kept as short as possible, particularly in inflammatory myositis, because one of the major side effects of longterm use of cortisone is muscle shrinkage and fat accumulation, which in itself can make muscles weak.

I decided to try the very latest in treatment options, which is *azathioprine*, another anti-inflammatory drug, added to intravenous *immunoglobulin* (IVIG), pooled antibodies from another source (see chapter 4). Fortunately, this proved a good combination. Vicki began to improve immediately, and within a few weeks her strength began to return. She had been ill for so long and unable to do so many things that she was astounded with her new-found power.

After several weeks in the hospital, Vicki was discharged. She remained on the medication and began seeing a physical therapist. She has since had to endure months of physical therapy to get back her strength, but she knows, particularly because of her experience as a dancer, that she is rebuilding her muscles, the largest single organ of the body (other than the skin). With the muscles, improvement is always gradual and sometimes painfully slow. She also is aware that she may need to be on medication for the rest of her life.

But then again, she may not. I have seen some young people—a few of them athletes—who progress in their disease to total weakness, requiring a wheelchair, and then, like Lazarus, rise to live a new and strong life. Other patients I have had remain debilitated for many years and never get back to normal. People are all different, even in their recovery, and I cannot predict who will have the best outcome. This is why I am always cautious in my expectations, and I share my caution with my patients.

When I suggested to Vicki on one of her recent office visits that it was realistic to expect that her dancing days might be behind her, she disagreed vehemently. She continues to insist that she will dance again. With that kind of determination, and knowing this ballerina as I do, I have a feeling she will prove me wrong. I sincerely hope she does.

CHAPTER SEVENTEEN

RHEUMATOID ARTHRITIS

~

Like Swimming through a Bowl of Jell-O

W HEN I FIRST met Rhonda, she and her family had just returned from a fall camping trip in the Rocky Mountains. Rhonda is a classic example of an out-doorswoman. Strong and fit, she loves to hike, rock climb, and camp out. Every year she gathers up her accountant husband and two young sons, ages nine and eleven, and the family takes a three-day trip into the wilderness, or as much of a wilderness as you can find, four trail-hours out from a plush Ralph Lauren–inspired hunting lodge. Rhonda is the only one who gets excited about these trips. Her husband would much prefer to be in the lodge watching the Giants play football. As for the boys, "Well," she said later one afternoon, "neither of them has looked up from his Game Boy in two months— need I say more?"

On the second day into the trip, the family woke to very cold weather, and Rhonda found it exceedingly difficult to warm herself. By evening, she had developed a total body chill. "I couldn't shake it," she told me, "and I wondered why I was the only one who was so cold. Finally, wearing two pairs of socks, my husband's gloves, and anything I could find to cover myself with, I fell asleep. The next morning there was frost on the ground inside our tent, and I couldn't get out of my sleeping bag. Every move felt as if someone was banging on my joints with a hammer. I knew something was wrong, and I figured it was Lyme disease because I had seen a whole host of deer the day before. But no ticks were on my body. Believe me, we looked. At that point, it didn't matter. I just wanted to get out of those godforsaken woods and back to the lodge."

"How did you manage that?" I asked.

"Well, first the boys built a fire near the tent. Then, after a few hours, four ibuprofen tablets, and a lot of stretching, the pains subsided so I was able to walk, though not easily. They all took turns helping me. It took forever to get back to the lodge, but I did it."

"And once you got there? How did you feel?"

"Would that be before or after the three brandies?"

Rhonda was experiencing the acute phase of rheumatoid arthritis. Though she did not know it at the time, the rapid onset of the terrible pain and incapacitating stiffness was indeed quite serious. A cold autumn morning in the middle of the damp woods is certainly no place to have this happen (not that there is an ideal place). Her concerns about Lyme disease were valid, since the deer ticks that carry it are prevalent in the north woods, and the illness epidemic in the summer months. But symptoms of Lyme do not appear that fast, and Lyme disease usually begins with a rash, which she did not have.

Rhonda had seen her family physician first, and I met her several days after she returned from the disastrous camping trip. Before our meeting, she had taken a midnight tour of the Internet and arrived armed with a legal pad full of questions and a detailed list of her symptoms, which I always appreciate. The presence of morning stiffness and the location of her joint pains practically headlined rheumatoid arthritis, particularly because the joint pains were on both sides of her body at the same time, which is one of the requisites for diagnosis of this disease. In cases of true RA, if one knee is affected, the other one must always be affected as well. Morning stiffness that occurs for at least one hour or more, which she had, also is characteristic.

I did not feel comfortable telling her my suspicions on the spot because so many illnesses resemble rheumatoid arthritis but are not autoimmune-related, and it is necessary to rule these out first. For example, Lyme disease, which has as its symptoms low fever, joint pain, and fatigue, is a very close mimic of RA. The same symptoms exist with *parvovirus* infection which, when it affects children, is known as *Fifth's disease* or *slapped cheek syndrome* (for its associated bright-red coloring that appears across the cheeks). Parvovirus can cause significant arthritis or a special kind of anemia in adults. *Ehrlichiosis,* a condition involving an unusual bacterium that lives within certain parts of the white cell, is another mimic of RA and, like Lyme disease, is transmitted by ticks. (When I hike through the woods these days, I wear clothing with long sleeves and long pants and on return, I always look for ticks on my trusty hounds, the Velts, otherwise known as "Teddy" and "Rosie.") So when looking for RA in a patient, we always have to look beyond it. Unfortunately, no single test exists that can confirm this diagnosis.

What Is Rheumatoid Arthritis?

Rheumatoid arthritis is a chronic autoimmune disorder in which the immune system attacks the joints and surrounding tissues. It is the most prevalent of the autoimmune diseases, striking more than 2.5 million people in this country, 80 percent of whom are women. This complicated illness expresses itself in many ways. For example, RA can be exclusively articular, meaning it involves only the joints, or it can be extra-articular, in which case it can also affect the peripheral nerves, lungs, muscles, heart, and blood-vessel walls. There are even some syndromes within the disease itself. *Palindromic rheumatism* is one such variant of RA, in which patients experience pain that reaches peak intensity within a few hours and then the pain resolves again within an identical number of hours. In other words, the symptoms come and go like a palindrome. (Remember the palindrome: "Madam, I'm Adam"?)

Felty's syndrome is another RA-associated disease, in which the white cells drop, fever begins, and the spleen enlarges to the size of a football. Felty's syndrome is a very severe type of RA and the arthritis-associated pain is very bad. But it is not permanent. I treat these patients aggressively with Remicade, methotrexate, or Enbrel.

Generally, with continuous treatment, the spleen returns to standard size, the white cells come back to normal, and the symptoms resolve. Felty's may be a form of rheumatoid vasculitis.

▷ *The Disease Process*

The process of RA almost always follows this course: After the immune system recognizes what it believes is an antigen in the joint capsule, T cells travel to the synovium, a layer of cells that cover the joint (like Aunt Frieda's plastic-wrapped couch) and, once there, cause an immune reaction that precipitates inflammation, swelling, and pain. During the inflammation process, the cells grow and divide, making the normally thin synovium thick, resulting in a swollen joint or joints. In addition, a benign tumor called a *pannus* forms in and around the joint. The pannus, which does not appear with any other form of arthritis, looks like the original blob of movie fame; the one that rolled around engulfing everything in sight. While this is not a terribly scientific description, it is the best visual I can offer because it describes precisely how rheumatoid arthritis proceeds. The pannus encircles the cartilage and bone of the joint and secretes chemicals that begin to eat away at the bone's surface. When the cells begin to invade the cartilage and bone within the joint, the surrounding muscles, ligaments, and tendons become weak and are unable to function normally, leading to pain and deformity. As a buildup of scar tissue replaces the damaged tissue, the spaces in the joints narrow and movement becomes limited. A pannus can be removed surgically, but it is a very difficult operation and in the end, the pannus (like the blob) may reappear. If it recurs, it does so to a far lesser degree than its original state. Approximately 25 percent of people with RA will develop rheumatoid nodules, or bumps under the skin, which are found close to the joints.

Some people with RA experience only mild joint stiffness, interrupted by periodic inflammatory flareups. In others, however, symptoms are persistent and worsen over time, causing deformities of the hands and feet. In very severe cases, rheumatoid arthritis also can affect the heart, lungs, muscles, and skin. Joint damage generally begins in the first year or two after the onset of disease. A number of doctors hold to the notion that RA exists for a finite amount of time and then symptoms disappear forever, but I am not so sure. As I said earlier, so many conditions mimic RA that I believe it is likely those patients in whom symptoms disappeared simply did not have genuine RA to begin with.

Disease Patterns

RA is both similar to and different from the other autoimmune diseases. It resembles them in that symptoms vary from one person to the next. As with lupus and multiple sclerosis, symptoms of RA can follow two courses: They can come and go, with flares occurring on occasion, or they can be linear (or progressive), meaning that the disease is always evident and progresses more slowly. Also, like many other autoimmune diseases, RA is multisystemic, with the ability to affect all body organs and tissues, including the eye, lungs, or skin. Actually, RA can strike almost anywhere and leave its mark. For example, it can exist alongside vasculitis (see chapter 9), which results in inflammation of the blood vessels. When the eyes are affected, perforation from rheumatoid nodules can occur on the surface of the eyeball, causing loss of vision that can sometimes be permanent. When the lungs are involved, shortness of breath results.

What makes rheumatoid arthritis different from most of the other autoimmune diseases is its most prominent antibody, called *rheumatoid factor*. Rheumatoid factor is an antibody that targets other antibodies. It is essentially an anti-antibody. But here is the kicker: If, in our efforts to diagnose RA, we identify rheumatoid factor, we still cannot say for certain that the patient has RA, for a couple of reasons. First, rheumatoid factor is found in many other conditions, such as infections (including rheumatic fever and other blood infections caused by strep bacteria) and conditions such as cirrhosis of the liver or kidney disease. It is also found in Sjögren's syndrome, lupus, or rheumatic fever, to name a few. But rheumatoid factor, like ANA (antinuclear antibodies), is rarely specific to any autoimmune disease. As I have mentioned, "specific" means that if the antibody is found in a blood test, you can be certain the disease exists, and if it is not found, the disease does not exist. I wish it were that easy with RA, but it is not. Only 60 percent of RA patients are positive for rheumatoid factor antibodies.

Rheumatoid Arthritis versus Osteoarthritis

I want to note the specific distinctions between rheumatoid arthritis and osteoarthritis (degenerative arthritis), the most common form of arthritis. First, osteoarthritis is not an autoimmune disease. Second, in people with RA, the joint involvement is usually symmetrical, while in osteoarthritis it usually is not. In addition, the affected joints in the fingers of people with RA are the ones nearest the palm of the hand, as opposed to the ones at the fingertips, which are usually affected first in osteoarthritis. Finally, the more common osteoarthritis affects only the musculoskeletal system, whereas RA can afflict any part of the body including, as described above, the eyes, lungs, heart, and blood vessels. Unfortunately, neither of these diseases is curable.

Causes of Rheumatoid Arthritis

Finding a cause of RA is proving to be as difficult as finding the cause of cancer. Over the last fifty years, investigators have identified everything from malaria to viruses as a cause of RA, but none has proven to be the true source. It is known that certain genes that play a role in the immune system are associated with the tendency to develop RA, but some people with RA do not have these genes, and others who have them never develop the disease. This suggests that genetic makeup, while important to the story, is not the whole story. It is also clear that more than one gene is involved in determining whether a person will develop RA and how severe the disease will become.

Many scientists charge the environment with triggering the disease process in people whose genetic makeup renders them susceptible to

RA. An infectious agent, such as a virus or bacterium, also appears to be a likely culprit, but for now, we do not know which agent it is. With four times as many women as men suffering from rheumatoid arthritis, it appears that hormonal factors also may be involved. Personally, I believe that this disease is caused by infection, one that uses an elusive new mechanism. I also believe RA may be a disease with many causes. The sad truth is, for all the scientific research that has transpired, we are no closer to understanding the cause of this malady than we were thirty years ago.

Diagnosing Rheumatoid Arthritis

Because symptoms are always symmetrical, it might seem that diagnosing RA would be easier than diagnosing most other autoimmune diseases, but it is not the case. Too many other factors come into play, and with no single test to rely on that might confirm the disease, I always begin a workup in a similar way. With Rhonda, I started by taking her history, and followed with a physical examination and a number of reliable tests.

▷ History

Rhonda had not yet experienced the severe fatigue, pain, or fever that most RA patients describe at the very beginning of their disease. Had she done so, I would have asked her, as I do with all my patients, to get a bit more specific. For example, I ask a likely RA patient: "When you wake up in the morning, swing your legs over the side of the bed, and stand up with your weight on your feet, does it feel like you're walking on shards of broken glass?" If the answer is a resounding "Yes," I am ready to lay odds that the patient has rheumatoid arthritis. It is that painful, which is no surprise when you consider what is going on inside those feet. The bones are literally being chewed. Enzymes are digesting the ligaments, the tendons, the cartilage, and the bone itself. Then there is the other telltale sign—morning stiffness that lasts more than thirty minutes. Patients say it feels like they are swimming through a big bowl of Jell-O, or that the air around them feels thick and heavy. That is how difficult it is to move. Some have three hours of stiffness, others have twelve. As if that is not bad enough, the symptoms come on suddenly for most patients, as they did with Rhonda. One minute she felt fine, and suddenly all hell broke loose.

▷ *Physical Examination*

With Rhonda in my examining room, I performed the exercises I deem essential to confirm a diagnosis of rheumatoid arthritis. First, I looked for certain characteristics of the disease, such as tender and swollen joints, generally in the wrists and the finger joints nearest the palm and the knees, feet, toes, and bottoms of the feet nearest the toes. I looked for a symmetrical pattern to the affected areas and for the presence of nodules, or little bumps, on the tendons which go down the arm or the Achilles tendons behind the ankles. These *rheumatoid nodules* can arise in any part of the body, from the lungs to the heart, and are very important to the overall outcome of the disease. Nodules have gained in importance in the examination because recent studies show that the patients with rheumatoid nodules respond better to the disease-modifying drugs—also known as DMARDs—that are discussed later in the chapter.

I observed that Rhonda's joints were swollen and that she had a limited range of motion. When I pressed on a few of the joints (not my favorite thing to do), it caused exquisite pain, an unmistakable telltale sign of inflammation. That, combined with the symmetrical pattern of her swollen joints, let me know that I was still going in the right direction. It was time for some additional testing.

▷ *X-ray*

When X-raying a patient's hands and wrists, I look for any signs of bone loss caused by inflammation in the joint space. The indication in early disease is actually a bleaching or blanching of the bone structure around the joints. This is called *reabsorption*, or technically speaking, *periarticular osteopenia*, and it is a telltale sign of RA. Osteopenia, or thinning of the bone mass itself, is characteristic of rheumatoid arthritis but is also found in many women who do not have this disease. An X-ray of Rhonda's hands and wrists showed not only bleached bones, but also barely perceptible erosions of the joint margins. In short: Rhonda's X-ray was indicative of RA, but not specific to it. As in so many of the autoimmune diseases, each of the diagnostic tests that we use plays an important role, but because so few are definitive, their value is as part of an aggregate that tells the diagnostic story. Now that I knew Rhonda had the primary signs of RA, I planned to go further in my search for scientific evidence of the disease.

▷ Laboratory Tests

In the blood tests I ordered for Rhonda, I looked for antibody or autoimmune proteins in her blood and for rheumatoid factor, although, as I said earlier, the latter is not found in all people with RA. In fact, very few antibodies are found in the blood of patients with RA. When rheumatoid factor is not present, the condition is called *sero negative* rheumatoid arthritis, but it is RA nevertheless. Making the diagnosis without the antibodies to back you up is still a crap shoot for most of us, since we often have to begin therapy in the blind faith that our diagnosis is the correct one.

Treating Rheumatoid Arthritis

Of course, it would be better if there were no need for such treatment at all, but I almost want to say it is a pleasure these days to treat patients with rheumatoid arthritis. Treating RA is so much easier than it used to be because there are so many new and exciting options to offer my patients. Of course, I am still a fan of the old mainstays: medication and a good balance between exercise and rest. Let us address these two now. *Exercise*, such as swimming and walking, is essential to preserve joint mobility and flexibility, but I suggest you only do so to the degree that it is comfortable. Stop at the first sign of pain. *Rest* is equally important, and short rest breaks are more helpful than a lot of time spent in bed. Consider stress reduction as well. Although we cannot say that stress causes RA, I do know from experience that it can make living with the disease more difficult and may also affect the amount of pain a person feels.

▷ *Gold*

Before I discuss RA medications, I want to say a word here about gold. Many years ago, gold was all the rage for treatment of RA. I still do not understand precisely how it works, but for some, it does appear to alleviate the pain and symptoms and get rid of the erosive disease. When treating a patient with gold, the precious metal is put into a liquid solution and injected into the patient once a week. A single shot is relatively inexpensive; it cost only a few dollars when last I checked, which I admit was some time ago. The reason I stopped using gold as a treatment is that there are so many better medications available today, and I do not like its side effects. One of the bad side effects of gold treatment is *proteinurea,* or protein in the urine. This condition develops when the kidney membranes, the filtration mechanism, are negatively affected by the gold. As a result, the protein, instead of being held back by the filter, spills into the urine. Proteinurea can ultimately lead to kidney disease. When gold is used as therapy for RA, the treating physician must keep a careful record of how much gold has been given, because the body can tolerate only a specific amount before its use becomes counterproductive.

▷ *Drugs*

The bounty of new and sophisticated drugs that have come along in the past thirty years have dramatically changed the face of RA treatment. People who could not brush their hair or work a zipper are able to work, exercise, and lead relatively normal lives, thanks to the research and development of these new drugs. Aspirin and its derivatives were the first early medications offered to attack the pain of RA because they diminished the inflammatory process—the cause of painful, red, and immobile joints. These drugs were classified as nonsteroidal anti-inflammatories (NSAIDs). But the problems with these drugs were the side effects people suffered in order to get pain relief. These comprise a class of drugs called COX or cyclooxygenase inhibitors, which are like very specific super-aspirins that get rid of pain and inflammation. Aspirin, Naprosyn, Meclomen, and Indocin are the most popular of these nonspecific agents. Now, a more specific version of these COX inhibitors—called COX2—are so selective as to allow pain relief without the side effects. These include drugs like Celebrex. These and all drugs for RA are discussed in full detail in chapter 19.

Another wonderful advance in treating rheumatoid arthritis is the advent of drugs called *DMARDs*, or disease-modifying arthritis-related drugs, which do not treat the symptoms, but rather treat the disease process. The chemotherapeutic drugs such as methotrexate, hydroxychloroquine, and Imuran are examples of DMARDs that I give to patients early in the game to prevent the destruction of bone and joints.

▷ *Biological Response Modifiers: The New New Thing*

As terrific as it is to be able to relieve pain and prevent the inexorable destruction of joints, today the big excitement is in the *biological response modifiers*. This new approach to RA is designed to interrupt the work of cytokines, the communications molecules. If we block these message-carrying molecules—cytokines, like tumor necrosis factor (TNF), and chemokines—we can block the messages and ultimately abort or at least slow down the disease process. TNF is a fundamental cytokine that does amazing things within the body. But in biology, as in life, everything is a trade-off. For example, by blocking TNF, the patient will generally feel better as joint pains subside and the erosions go away. But some negative effects also can occur, although they are very rare. For example, I have heard that some patients have developed demyelination—a stripping of the covering of the nerve sheath—although I have never seen it, and there is a danger of very serious bacterial infection. This probably has to do with the fact that some natural defenses against the bacteria are inhibited with the TNF. In any case, a person who is infected with a bacterium while on these drugs would require very aggressive treatment with antibiotics.

Blocking cytokines, although very effective, is not to be taken lightly. Still, I have patients on these drugs who could not move several years ago and who are now running marathons. The cytokine inhibitors, which include Enbrel, Remicade, and Humira, may not represent a cure, but they have certainly allowed my patients to conduct themselves as though they do not even have a disease.

▷ *Pregnancy*

Pregnancy is a very special state that challenges the already complicated female physiognomy. During this most miraculous time, the body changes everything from the volume of blood that goes to the heart to the number of antibody molecules that are designed to protect the fetus. For a pregnant woman with rheumatoid arthritis, these changes become immeasurably more complicated. Certain substances in the blood of pregnant women cause the complete, if temporary, amelioration of pain and discomfort in the majority of women with RA, and many RA sufferers look forward to pregnancy for that reason. Those substances include molecules such as pregnancy-associated glycoprotein, antibody isotype (different forms), and steroid hormones.

To reinforce the idea that something during pregnancy temporarily cures rheumatoid arthritis, investigators a few years ago suggested that the incidence of RA in women was dropping due to the increased use of birth control pills, specifically those that contained a lot of estrogen. Naturally, some physicians started to prescribe estrogen-containing tablets as oral contraceptives to their RA patients, but it had no effect on the disease. Just which cytokines or other agents in the blood of pregnant women mitigate this disease for a limited period continues to remain a mystery. If we could just figure out what message is being given to the pregnant woman, and when and why, we might be able to cure this and many other rheumatic diseases.

Here is the not-so-good news: After delivery of the baby, RA generally comes back with a vengeance.

Rhonda's Story, Continued

Disease progression is always a significant issue of concern to any patient with RA. Rhonda remembered that her late grandmother had this condition and was confined to a wheelchair. She could not walk or grasp very well with her hands. The grandmother had died young from her disease, at age sixty-two, so naturally Rhonda was concerned that it might turn out the same way for her. But she will never be like her grandmother, because she is being treated with the spectacular new drugs that were not available when her grandmother was alive. Her grandmother simply lived at the wrong time.

In the past twenty years, we have learned much about the cytokine-related communication networks, the inflammatory processes, and most important, the immune system itself, knowledge that has put us in the forefront of research in certain diseases, including rheumatoid arthritis. Moreover, it seems that every month at one scientific meeting or another, a new drug is discussed that may change the course of the disease. It is because of these new and amazing agents that I keep assuring Rhonda, "This is not your grandmother's disease." Actually, it is and it is not. The disease is the same, but that is *all* that is. The treatment is so radically improved that nothing else can be compared.

CHAPTER EIGHTEEN

FIBROMYALGIA, CHRONIC FATIGUE SYNDROME, AND SILICONE IMPLANT SYNDROME

⁓

The Mystery Diseases

ALTHOUGH FIBROMYALGIA AND chronic fatigue syndrome (CFS)—and for that matter, silicone-implant-induced disease, if it exists—are not technically considered autoimmune diseases, I have included these subjects in this book because they are so closely associated with many of the autoimmune diseases. I have linked them together in this chapter because they all exemplify what I consider to be mystery diseases—right up there with Gulf War syndrome and Tokyo subway disease—for which there is no known diagnosis, cause, or treatment.

Fibromyalgia

I believe that fibromyalgia is a real disease, if not necessarily autoimmune, although many of my colleagues do not agree. While some are at a loss to explain fibromyalgia, others consider it a psychiatric problem and refuse to see patients who claim to have the malady. I confess that I also used to question its existence, but since becoming an autoimmunologist, I have seen hundreds of women with fibromyalgia, and I find it hard to believe that each of them consulted one another or a textbook before visiting me. Yet that's how remarkably similar their symptoms are.

Fibromyalgia is an illness of chronic pain that involves the muscles and multiple tender points in localized areas, as listed below. Patients with fibromyalgia also describe bouts of fluid retention, bloating, abdominal pain, cold intolerance, dizziness, jaw pain, swelling, numbness and tingling, depression, and anxiety. Others have stiffness, which leads them to believe their problems are arthritis-related. Some are so debilitated by their symptoms that they lose their appetite, and many suffer from depression and insomnia. In fact, fibromyalgia is so often associated with a lack of sleep that many physicians refer to it as primarily a sleep disorder.

No one knows what triggers fibromyalgia, although there are many theories. I have heard everything from an injury or trauma that affects the central nervous system, to changes in muscle metabolism that decrease blood flow and lead to fatigue. I have also heard the condition blamed on a viral infection, although to date no specific virus has been identified. We clearly see more of this kind of disease after events like September 11, which reinforces my belief that the psyche, while not responsible, is inextricably involved and that fibromyalgia is definitely stress-related. An emotional event, such as a divorce, or even experiencing so simple a thing as a missed airplane flight can bring on a painful episode of fibromyalgia.

According to the American College of Rheumatology (ACR), fibromyalgia currently affects 3 to 6 million Americans. Like most autoimmune diseases, it occurs primarily in women of childbearing age, but men, children, and the elderly can be affected. Why women are affected more often than men is unclear, but it may have to do with hormones, as described in chapter 2.

▷ *Diagnosing Fibromyalgia*

Because of the increasing reports of cases, in 1990 the ACR officially recognized fibromyalgia as a disease and devised a set of guidelines for a clinical diagnosis. The criteria indicate that the patient should have widespread pain for three months or more on both sides of the body. The ACR has identified eighteen tender points, which consist of either the right or left sides of nine areas of the body. Commonly referred to as "trigger points," a patient must have eleven or more of them in order to fit the diagnosis of fibromyalgia. To identify true involvement of a trigger point, the physician presses down on the tender area with about four kilograms of digital pressure to bring on pain in the tender areas. This amount of pressure is about enough to blanch a thumbnail, that is, to turn the fingernail white when pressing down. (Sometimes I feel these criteria are so primitive as to feed the natural doubts of many of my colleagues, as well as my own.) The amount of pain these patients feel when I touch a trigger point is, of course, subjective. But I have my own barometer, which I have termed the "chandelier sign." (You press on the trigger point and the patient hits the chandelier.)

Here are the trigger points. Please note that these can be on the right or left sides of the following nine areas, and in some cases, are on both sides at the same time:

▷ Neck
▷ Shoulders
▷ Chest
▷ Rib cage
▷ Thighs
▷ Lower back
▷ Knees
▷ Arms (elbows)
▷ Buttocks

Fibromyalgia is often diagnosed as secondary to autoimmune disease. As if this disease were not bad enough on its own, picture what these symptoms, feeling lousy, suffering from insomnia or constipation, must be like alongside a disease such as lupus or Sjögren's syndrome, polymyositis, vasculitis, or rheumatoid arthritis. In fact, fibromyalgia is reported in about 25 percent of patients with lupus, 25 percent of patients with RA, and 50 percent of patients with Sjögren's syndrome. In some cases of Sjögren's syndrome, fibromyalgia is the first symptom to appear.

▷ *Treating Fibromyalgia*

The treatment of fibromyalgia in its primary form—when it is unconnected to another disease—varies from patient to patient and doctor to doctor. Because there is no antibody that we know of for this disease, there is no role for immunosuppression in fibromyalgia. Treating generalized pain with nonaddictive pain drugs and prescribing antidepressants to aid sleep are the mainstays of therapy. I personally believe, although not everyone agrees, that fibromyalgia is a sleep disorder, and sleep disorders are best treated by having the patient sleep. The first question I ask a fibromyalgia patient is, Do you sleep? Inevitably, they say "No." They say the pain keeps them awake and, if they do fall asleep, wakes them up many times during the night. The tricyclic (antidepressant) taken about an hour before bed lets people go into a deeper REM sleep. I also put patients on analgesic drugs such as Tylenol, Darvon, or Tramadol. Pain in a specific muscle is best treated with passive stretching and local anesthetics applied directly to the offending trigger point.

Many patients report relief with an integrative therapy plan that combines, for example, physical therapy with relaxation, biofeedback, and/or medication as prescribed by a physician. I have no qualms with any of the complementry therapies as long as they are done with the knowldege of the treating physician. (See chapter 20 for a list of complementary treatments.)

I find that aerobic exercises such as walking and swimming are wonderful additions to fibromyalgia treatment. In some cases, if need be, psychological counseling can help, although I am not sure a psychologist is warranted except perhaps to help the person get through the early stages of the disease.

A major issue with diagnosing and treating fibromyalgia when it occurs with other diseases is that some physicians merge its symptoms and signs with the other disease and treat the patient with steroids or other medications in an effort to treat the underlying autoimmune disease. I have seen them give a steroid dose as high as 100 milligrams, and still be faced with a patient in persistent pain. The outcome is a patient who is being overtreated, who cannot sleep, who is hurting all over, and who has two diseases, one of which is not being addressed. This is a real problem. And this is where the specialist comes in, because a good one can differentiate between fibromyalgia and an autoimmune disease and not combine the two into one illness.

Chronic Fatigue Syndrome

Chronic fatigue syndrome (CFS) is a complex condition characterized by profound exhaustion that is not improved by bed rest and that can get worse with physical activity. It is a real problem for many young women (and men) who go from doctor to doctor, feeling awful and seeking a cure. Part of the issue with this condition is that the symptoms are nonspecific and subjective. For example, the following symptoms can all be associated with CFS, but experiencing them does not necessarily indicate the presence of the disease:

▷ Weakness
▷ Flulike symptoms
▷ Generalized pain
▷ Insomnia
▷ Difficulty with concentration or memory
▷ Sore throat
▷ Tender lymph nodes
▷ Muscle pain
▷ Multijoint pain without swelling or redness
▷ Headaches
▷ Unrefreshing sleep

Despite a significant amount of research, the source of this condition eludes us. I believe that CFS may in fact have multiple origins. Viruses, other infectious agents, or toxins might contribute to some but not all cases. CFS may be caused in part by a breakdown somewhere in the immune system, such as too many or too few cytokines, or an altered capacity of certain immune functions. One intriguing hypothesis is that a triggering event, such as stress or a viral infection, may lead to the chronic expression of cytokines and then to CFS. Administration of some cytokines in therapeutic doses is known to cause fatigue, but no characteristic pattern of chronic cytokine secretion has ever been identified in CFS patients.

▷ Diagnosing Chronic Fatigue Syndrome

It is important to understand that because of the amorphous nature of this disease, making a diagnosis is highly subjective. As with most medical conditions, the first step in diagnosing CFS is obtaining a detailed medical history and performing a complete physical examination. I order laboratory tests on all my patients to see if there are any other possible causes of illness. Because many illnesses have incapacitating fatigue as a symptom, I try to exclude other known and sometimes treatable conditions. If no cause for the symptoms is identified, and my patient exhibits at least three or four of the symptoms listed above for three months, I will probably render a diagnosis of CFS.

▷ Clinical Course of Chronic Fatigue Syndrome

CFS patients generally alternate between periods of illness and relative well-being. At the onset of illness, the most commonly reported symptoms are sore throat, fever, muscle pain, and muscle weakness. As the illness progresses, muscle pain and forgetfulness increase, and the reporting of depression appears to decrease. The actual percentage of patients who recover from CFS is unknown, and even the definition of what should be considered recovery is subject to debate. Some patients recuperate to the point that they can resume work and other activities, but continue to experience various or periodic CFS symptoms. Some patients recover completely with time, and others, I am sorry to say, grow progressively worse. I have never known of anyone who died from this problem, but many have become so debilitated as to call it a "living death."

▷ Treating Chronic Fatigue Syndrome

A variety of therapeutic approaches may benefit patients with CFS, but because no cause has been identified, treatment is directed at relief of symptoms and returning a patient to her earlier level of function and well-being. When CFS exists with other autoimmune diseases, I always take into consideration the treatment for these diseases before prescribing a therapeutic regimen for the CFS. In most cases, I suggest lifestyle changes that work for everyone. For example, physical activity is known to be helpful for physical and emotional well-being, although a key consideration for patients with CFS is to know how much to do, when to do it, and when to stop. It is important for anyone with CFS to avoid increasing the level of fatigue. I also suggest to my patients that even though they may be feeling better, they should still take it easy, because excessive activity can bring on a relapse.

A manageable daily routine includes modest regular exercise such as walking and swimming. In cases where patients have accompanying autoimmune disease, it is helpful if an early exercise program can be supervised by a knowledgeable health-care provider or physical therapist. Some patients feel they are helped by complementary therapeutic methods such as massage therapy, acupuncture, self-hypnosis, or biofeedback (see chapter 20).

Currently, investigators are looking at cytokine levels in the brain and in the peripheral blood supply to see if there are differences between those who are not fatigued and those who are, and how those differences play out. (The cytokine changes may be the cause of chronic fatigue syndrome and low-grade fever.) But we are still in the early days in this field, and unfortunately not likely to see much in the way of results of such investigations for many years. Much of this ongoing research is fraught with criticism both from within the professional community, who feel that it is a waste of time, and from outside the community from insurance groups and HMOs that will not reimburse studies or physician time. The field is so riddled with nonscientific guessing and presumption—for example: exposure to hair dye or diet soda will lead to CFS—that it is all but impossible to do unbiased research in this area. I am hopeful, though, that perhaps soon some discovery will help us understand this grievous malady.

Silicone Implant Syndrome

One of the hot medical stories of the 1990s was silicone breast implants, their connection to many autoimmune diseases, and the litigious furor sparked by the association. Most particularly, silicone implants were linked to chronic fatigue syndrome and fibromyalgia. I have labeled this condition *silicone implant syndrome.*

Silicone was introduced as an inert substance for breast enhancement back in the 1940s. Since that time, there have been thousands of conflicting reports on whether silicone placed in the body could affect the body's physiology. In 1992, the implants were taken off the market because of the many reports coming from women who claimed to have developed implant-related illnesses. According to a report in the *New York Times,* in the eleven-year period following the removal of the implants from the market, hundreds of thousands of women sued the manufacturers of these devices. Despite the fact that all evidence pointed to the contrary, many women were awarded large sums of money and, today, of the ten companies that made implants, only one—Inamed—is still in the business.

Because this is such a big issue, to be fair, I feel I should report on both sides of the argument. I have heard anecdotally that many patients who had implants developed hypergammaglobulinemia, a sign of super-antibody production. I have heard about women who have developed rheumatoid arthritis, mixed connective tissue disease (a form of scleroderma), and lupus. Are these reports true? I cannot say yes or no because I have not examined all these women, nor have I been privy to their records. On the other hand, as a scientist, my choice is to go with the scientific evidence, which says there is *no* causal relationship.

What exactly does silicone do that could possibly make it a precursor to autoimmune disease? Silicone could act as an adjuvant, a material that actually boosts the immune system. For example, many pharmaceutical companies add adjuvants to vaccines to strengthen the immune response to a foreign substance. Tetanus toxoid is an example of a substance given with an adjuvant. The people who believe an implant makes an immune response worse are saying that the silicone is the adjuvant that sets the immune system in search of an antigen.

According to many reports, silicone does produce antibodies, which may in fact be the way this whole debate started. Except the antibodies that are produced by silicone do not cause disease. Not all antibodies are disease-related. One study, for example, showed that silicone implants produced antithyroid antibodies and antibodies to cow collagen (a substance that is similar to the collagen found within human tissues). However, none of the patients with either thyroid antibodies or cow collagen antibodies developed disease of the thyroid or of the skin and other connective tissues. (Can people really have cow collagen antibodies? Yes, people can make antibodies to just about anything that their immune systems consider unusual, even the collagen from cows. If the conditions are right, people can make antibodies to milk protein, soy, or just about anything that goes down the esophagus.) In fact, the allergists believe that some of this aberrant antibody formation, while innocuous most of the time, can result in certain food allergies.

I suspect there will always be controversy surrounding silicone breast implants, and emotions will continue to run high, particularly because of the deeper issues. First, women want to look as good as they can, and many believe the answer lies in breast augmentation. Saline implants are available, but they feel different and cause different problems. But the greater issue is really the ability to reconstruct a breast after surgery for breast cancer. Once silicone implants became an option, women were devastated to learn they would have to give them up. Fortunately, that's all in the past. On October 15, 2003, after an eleven-year hiatus when silicone implants were not allowed on the market, the Food and Drug Administration cited their safety and recommended that women once again be granted access to them. The FDA determined that there is no causal relationship between silicone implants and *any* disease. Even so, at this writing, silicone implants are still not widely available.

PART THREE

Treatments

CHAPTER NINETEEN

DRUGS AND OTHER THERAPIES

Harnessing the Immune System

ECAUSE THERE IS as yet no cure for autoimmune disease, most treatment consists of alleviating the symptoms and slowing the immune system's destruction of the affected organs or tissues. New drugs for these purposes are being studied every day, and those deemed beneficial are released periodically. Today, many of these drugs are so good that they allow people with autoimmune disease to live quite normal lives. In fact, a great many reach remission, although even in remission, drugs must often be continued to ensure that the disease remains in check.

Medicine, as I have mentioned, is half art, half science, and, with a nod to Yogi Berra, half luck. This certainly holds true when it comes to treating autoimmune diseases, although treatment always requires an expert with experience to calculate the dosage of a drug or drugs, the duration of therapy, and simply to know what to use when, for what, on whom. This is one of those areas where it is critical to have a well-trained and proficient physician specialist. Doing so can mean the difference between a good and a bad outcome.

off

Experienced physicians can be found through a little research. I suggest calling a teaching hospital affiliated with a medical school or contacting such organizations as the Arthritis Foundation, the Autoimmune Disease Foundation, the Lupus Foundation, and the Sjögren's Foundation, to name a few. Actually, almost every autoimmune disease is connected with an association or a foundation, and they can be most helpful. See the appendix of helpful organizations for a full list.

In the earlier chapters, I briefly discussed the ways in which specific diseases are treated. This chapter provides more details about the pharmacological aspects of the medications physicians use to treat autoimmune diseases and explains why they work and what their side effects are. Following is an overview of the latest arsenal of drugs and treatments as we employ them today.

Diseases, Drugs, and the FDA

This may come as a surprise, but currently, most of the drugs that physicians use for autoimmune diseases are considered "off label," which means they are not approved for use in treating autoimmune diseases. Yes, you read correctly. The Food and Drug Administration (FDA) does not approve some of the drugs that I—and I speak here only for myself—use in my own work. Some of these drugs are still in clinical trials to determine their safety on humans. Others have been deemed safe for some diseases but are awaiting FDA approval for use in others. Many older drugs that are broadly employed have been used this way for many decades. That is, their safety has been established for one disease, and physicians use them for another. I believe that most patients understand and appreciate our limitations when it comes to using these drugs and the risks we take when we offer something that will not only increase the quality of their lives but prolong those lives as well. Patients only want to feel better, and fast. Unsurprisingly, that is also a physician's goal.

A caveat: Some of my patients who are desperate for a cure or are uncomfortable beyond my understanding will seek out remedies that are dangerous and unproven. Although I can clearly understand why they feel that way, it is up to me, and I take this very seriously, to explain how dangerous it is to go against conventional wisdom. I am not referring to the use of alternative or complementary therapies. Indeed, I agree with many of them and talk about them at length in the next chapter. Rather, I speak of following the advice of unfamiliar physicians—an M.D. after a name does not always signify an "expert"—as well as friends, family members, supermarket tabloids, or even the Internet. I tell my patients that following such advice can be tantamount to killing themselves while conducting their own clinical trials. So, when it comes to unauthorized treatments or drugs, please take a page from Nancy Reagan and just say "No."

Another caveat: Because everyone reacts differently to drugs, what works for one may not work for all. Also, drugs that may be heralded as the safest thing since baby oil may not be so safe when combined with other prescription or nonprescription, drugs, which is why it is imperative to consult your physician and read all warning labels.

At this writing, the drugs and treatments listed below are in use for managing various types of autoimmune diseases and syndromes. But before I venture into the world of pharmaceuticals, so that there is no confusion, I would like to say again: In the autoimmune diseases, other than the more recent biological response modifiers, which we spoke of in the chapter on rheumatoid arthritis, and which *do* affect immune function, there are very few therapeutic drugs that have an effect on the disease processes themselves. Most only relieve symptoms.

Nonsteroidal Anti-inflammatory Drugs: NSAIDs

As I have just mentioned, there are some drugs that we suspect will work for specific autoimmune diseases but have not been tested for those conditions. We use them because we know that symptoms such as pain from inflammation, which occurs in certain diseases, can be controlled with these drugs. One classification of these is the anti-inflammatory agents known as *nonsteroidal anti-inflammatory drugs,* NSAIDs (pronounced *en-sayeds*). NSAIDs act by inhibiting natural chemicals called *prostaglandins,* the principle hormones involved in inflammation. Actually, to be a purist about it, these drugs inhibit an enzyme or chemical activation molecule called a cyclooxygenase.

Since all of us get tongue-tied saying this word, we refer to the chemical as a COX.

NSAIDs are commonly used against injury, joint pain, fever, muscle aches, some rashes, and various forms of arthritis. As inflammation also can lead to pain, these drugs, by controlling inflammation, inadvertently control pain. However, they are not strictly referred to as analgesics or pain relievers. This drug classification includes both the old standbys and a newer generation. Aspirin is one of the older generations of prostaglandin inhibitors. The newer NSAIDs that we hear about daily on television—such as Celebrex—are an improvement over aspirin-type drugs because they block specific receptors. In other words, they are engineered to stick to the receptors on cells that ordinarily produce the prostaglandins. These hormones are directly involved in inflammation and pain. By blocking the receptor, the drug essentially blocks certain prostaglandins. The key word here is *certain,* but not all.

NSAIDs are used routinely all over the world. Until a few years ago, however, they caused an inordinate number of deaths—approximately 16,000 in 1997—from complications that included bowel perforation, ulcers, gastrointestinal bleeding, and kidney failure. The newer NSAIDs do not cause as much bleeding from stomach ulcers and are less likely to cause bowel and kidney problems, but they still can affect blood flow to the kidneys, the balance of minerals in the body, and, consequently, blood pressure. In other words, they are not perfect yet. Aspirin and COX1 and COX2 inhibitors are the most common types of NSAIDs.

▷ Aspirin

Aspirin is a classic anti-inflammatory drug that has been in constant use since 1889, when the Bayer Company in Germany patented it. It was actually the people at Bayer who came up with the name *aspirin.* The "A" stood for acetyl chloride, part of the compound that comprises the drug. The "spir" represented *Spiraea ulmaria,* the plant they derived the salicylic acid from, and the "in" was a then familiar name ending for medicines. Aspirin is a platelet inhibitor, and consequently a blood thinner, which makes it useful in preventing clots. It is believed that the drug protects those who take it regularly against strokes and heart attacks. It is still the best of the best when it comes to inhibiting prostaglandins, the rogues responsible for pain and inflammation.

Right now you are probably wondering: If aspirin does all this, why do we need anything else? The answer is a bit complicated. First of all, aspirin has side effects. Too much (or even a little) for too long a time can cause bleeding and stomach ulcers. This is because aspirin, in inhibiting all prostaglandins, inhibits the parts of prostaglandins that are protective as well as those that are destructive. In other words, aspirin does not select the kinds of prostaglandins it inhibits. Aspirin is the prototypical COX nonselective inhibitor. But there is now a new generation of drugs that *are* selective. These are the COX2 inhibitors.

▷ COX1 and COX2 Inhibitors

In an effort to create a more useful drug for patients who need relief from inflammation, but are also taking blood thinners, and for those with stomach and kidney problems, researchers have developed drugs that inhibit specific enzymes called *cyclooxygenases* (COX). There are two forms of COX enzymes: COX1 and COX2, both of which are active in the production of prostaglandins.

It is important to understand that prostaglandins are like Dr. Jeckyl and Mr. Hyde. That is, they have two sides: a good side and a bad one. The good side of prostaglandins, which is provided by the COX1 enzyme, protects the lining of the stomach, assures blood-vessel integrity, regulates blood pressure, and ensures the implantation of an egg in the uterus of a pregnant woman. The bad side is served by COX2, which is directly involved in inflammation, fever, and a host of other unfavorable symptoms. Until recently, all NSAIDs inhibited all COX enzymes, which meant that while they were restricting the bad prostaglandins, they restricted the good ones as well. In other words, while inhibiting COX2 kept inflammation and fever at bay, inhibiting COX1 at the same time compromised protection of the stomach lining and the blood vessels. Because this NSAID repressed both the good and the bad prostaglandins, the patient using it was left open to debilitating side effects. The drug was considered *nonselective* because it affected both COX enzymes. The nonselective NSAIDs include the old standbys such as aspirin, Indocin, Meclomen, and Naprosyn.

Several years ago, a search began to find a series of drugs that would be *selective*, that is, would inhibit only the COX2 enzyme, effectively removing the bad prostaglandins while keeping the good prostaglandins intact. The result is new, selective, COX2-blocking drugs that are protective of the body yet have the same effects of the nonselective NSAIDs. With these medications, we can avoid the bad effects of prostaglandin inhibition and get right to the root cause of inflammation. The selective drugs are *Celebrex* and some new ones like *Arcoxia*.

TABLE 1

COMMON DRUGS FOR INFLAMMATION: NONSTEROIDAL ANTI-INFLAMMATORIES (NSAIDs)

CLASS	POSITIVES	NEGATIVES
Aspirin	Reduces pain and inflammation. Has blood-thinning properties and thereby protects the heart and helps prevent stroke. Inexpensive.	Inhibits all COX enzymes. Causes stomach irritation in many people. Cannot be used with blood thinners.
COX1 and COX2 Inhibitors (Non-selective): Naprosyn Meclomen Indocin Voltaren	Provide great pain relief. Offer many choices.	Cause GI ulcers and indigestion in some patients and cannot be used with blood thinners. Moderately expensive.
COX2 Inhibitors (Selective): Celebrex Arcoxia	Provide great pain relief. Fairly safe on the stomach. Can be taken with blood-thinning medicine if patient is carefully watched.	May be associated with a slight increase of heart disease in some people. Known to cause an elevation of blood pressure. Still causes GI bleeding in some people. Very expensive.

Immunosuppressive Drugs

Some of the most remarkable drugs used in treating autoimmune diseases belong to the classification known as immunosupressives. These drugs, which vary in strength from mild to very potent, are designed to suppress the immune system in an effort to harness overactivity. They include cortisone and its derivatives, antimalarials, and chemotherapeutic compounds.

▷ Cortisone and Its Relatives

Cortisone, which is a steroid, is the pillar of the immunosupressives. In 1940, Dr. Phillip Hench discovered that this natural hormone could successfully be manufactured and used as an agent in the treatment of a number of autoimmune diseases. He eventually won the Nobel Prize for his discovery. Today, this medication is the major staple of early treatment of diseases such as lupus, Sjögren's syndrome, and vasculitis—diseases in which there is acute inflammation. Cortisone and its associated compounds *prednisone, dexamethasone,* and *methylprednisolone* weaken the immune system, and thereby reduce the immune response and ultimately inflammation. Cortisone must be prescribed properly, however. Too much can compromise the immune system, weakening it so much that an opportune infection can take over the body.

Because of cortisone, some patients with rheumatoid arthritis who had been unable to walk can now do so with little or no difficulty. Unfortunately, however, those patients who thought this drug was the Holy Grail did not realize the number of side effects that came with it. Cortisone can have consequences that are almost as devastating as the diseases that it is designed to alleviate. Bone loss, thinning skin, hair loss, irregular menses, fat accumulation at the nape of the neck and other parts of the body, increased appetite, and insomnia are all associated with cortisone, which is why I usually try to avoid prescribing it whenever I can. I am particularly careful about using it for chronic diseases, such as rheumatoid arthritis, because when cortisone frees a patient of pain, she is naturally reluctant to come off the drug. But in fact, as time goes on, patients sometimes require more to feel well, and this only promotes worse side effects.

All steroids must be used carefully and may never be discontinued abruptly. The only way to come off steroids is to taper them over a period of time, often months. The reason for this is directly connected to the adrenal glands, which produce cortisone naturally in our bodies. When cortisone is taken therapeutically for any period of time, the adrenal glands begin to slow down their own production of this hormone and eventually the glands begin to shrink. Coming off the drug slowly allows the adrenal glands to return to working order. This takes time, which is why the dose of drug is gradually lowered until the patient is off it entirely. Halting the drug abruptly carries side effects as well. The symptoms can be quite unpleasant and include weakness, tiredness, excessive sweating, salt retention, and a drastic rise in the potassium level.

While the body's natural cortisone is derived from the adrenal gland, most relatives of cortisone are synthetic. Cortisone is generally taken by mouth in pill form but can be administered intravenously as well. Methylprednisolone and dexamethasone are useful in such instances, such as during severe disease bouts, when a corticosteroid of higher potency is required. Sometimes steroids are put into ointments or creams and used topically for rashes and inflamed areas on the face or the torso. But because continued use of these agents in great concentration tends to cause shrinkage or atrophy of the skin, I caution against their overuse, particularly on sensitive areas such as the face.

▷ *Antimalarial Agents*

These drugs are excellent for use in a variety of autoimmune conditions, including lupus, antiphospholipid syndrome, and Sjögren's syndrome. They include *hydroxychloroquine* (Plaquenil) and *chloroquine* (Aralen), common medicines first used in the treatment of malaria, hence the name. The drugs, which are taken orally, are gentle immunosuppressive agents that lower cholesterol and thin the blood ever so slightly. There is evidence that hydroxychloroquine acts on the inner workings of the cell, although no one is really sure how it makes people with autoimmune disease better. There are almost no side effects from antimalarial agents except those affecting the eyes. Sometimes pigment is deposited in the retina, which can cause spots to appear in front of the eye and vision to diminish. Another side effect is a loss of sensation in the cornea, which causes an irritant-like feeling that can be very uncomfortable. These side effects occur in very few people, however, and are usually reversible, if detected early, by discontinuing the drug. Other reactions include itching, rash, and a bitter taste in the mouth.

The only requirement I have for patients taking hydroxychloroquine or any antimalarial drug, for that matter, is that they have an eye exam at the outset to provide a baseline and then every six months thereafter.

▷ *Chemotherapy*

The word chemotherapy is frightening to just about everyone because of its inextricable link to cancer. Actually, the term itself simply means "treated with chemicals." (In actuality, even taking an antibiotic is chemotherapy.) The mechanism behind most chemotherapy is to block cell division. Chemotherapy is given to patients with autoimmune disease in an effort to halt the rapidly dividing and highly damaging T cells. The more prolific the T cells, the stronger the autoimmune response. The problem is that chemotherapy, which is given systemically, acts on *all* cells. So, while slowing down the immune system's attacking action, it also slows down the immune system's protecting action, thus opening the body to infection or, worse, a malignancy down the road.

How does chemotherapy cause malignancy? These strong drugs can change the structure of the DNA or RNA or they can interfere with the cell's manufacture of vital materials, which is what happens when a cell's instructions get confused. This is just what we want to happen in the short term, but some of these drugs have lasting effects on the genetic makeup of the cells, which can surface later, and result in malignancy. Still, we are fortunate that we have such chemotherapeutic drugs available for times when the immune system is about to destroy a vital organ and urgent action is needed. In general, the dose of chemotherapy that is given for autoimmune disease is lower in strength and concentration than that prescribed for cancer.

The four most commonly used chemotherapeutic agents are methotrexate (Rheumatrex), leflunomide (Arava), azathioprine (Imuran), and cyclophosphamide (Cytoxan).

Methotrexate is a hallmark of therapy for autoimmune muscle diseases and other diseases, such as rheumatoid arthritis and lupus, because the once-a-week dose has very few major side effects. I am beginning to use methotrexate for a variety of autoimmune phenomena, not just the serious or life-threatening illnesses. This is because of its overall safety. However, the drug can damage the liver, so doctors must regularly test the liver function of patients who take it, and patients are cautioned to limit their alcohol consumption. Adverse effects can include sores in the mouth or a bronchitis-like cough, but these go away when the drug is discontinued. When a particularly damaging side effect occurs, the doctor may stop the drug and restart it later at a lower dose. Folic acid, when given simultaneously, can counter methotrexate-induced reactions such as oral blisters.

Leflunomide is another drug that is useful in the control of diseases like rheumatoid arthritis. I consider it an alternative to methotrexate, and it is very useful. The side effect profile is much like that of methotrexate, but it often lacks some of the untoward effects that patients on methotrexate complain about. I do not place patients taking leflunomide on folic acid. Like the others, this drug reduces disease activity and joint inflammation.

Azathioprine is another very useful agent in the treatment of the autoimmune diseases. As we have just seen, when a patient has autoimmune disease, her T cells are maturing, dividing, and turning over at tremendous rates. Azathioprine changes the structure of the DNA in these rapidly dividing cells and thereby slows down the immune response. But these agents can also transiently affect areas of the body that rely on critical cell division, such as the bone marrow and the liver. This drug can cause some degree of liver enzyme abnormality or even hepatitis if a patient is particularly sensitive. Azathioprine is also useful in major organ disease and as an agent that allows the doctor to lower the dose of cortisone. Hair loss may occur, but is usually reversible at the conclusion of treatment.

Cyclophosphamide is a strong chemotherapy drug that is used particularly for treatment of life-threatening forms of vasculitis, lupus, and other autoimmune diseases. It can be given intravenously or by mouth. It is not recommended for conditions such as autoimmune-related baldness (alopecia) or other mild manifestations of diseases, such as joint pains, rash, or even dry mucous membranes, as seen in Sjögren's syndrome. After a patient is given cyclophosphamide, she is given periodic blood tests to check on her white and red blood cell levels. The white cells should plummet after about seven to ten days of intravenous therapy, which is a measurable indication that the immune system is slowing down and that treatment is successful. Side effects include hair loss, mouth ulcers, bladder irritation, and inhibition of the bone marrow, leading to anemia. I reserve this drug for the serious situations where I need a really big gun.

I have given cyclophosphamide to many patients with success, including two members of the clergy, which prompted one of the local prelates to dub me the "Borgia of New York City." Unlike the Borgias, however, my victims live to a ripe old age, even after being intentionally poisoned by me.

▷ Disease-Modifying Antirheumatic Drugs

Agents such as those just listed that actually slow the progression of autoimmune disease are called DMARDs, which stands for disease-modifying antirheumatic drugs. Bone erosions, tendon weakness, fever, pain, and all of the other signs of acute disease can be stopped in their tracks by a DMARD. Until recently, doctors started treatment with painkillers and anti-inflammatory drugs and later added the DMARDs to control the illness. These days, physicians tend to think that the sooner the DMARD is added, the better the overall outcome for the patient. (Often, they are given during the first few weeks of symptoms.) Moreover, the standard for doctors is to use several DMARDs at the same time to achieve the closest-to-perfect result in the patient. Sometimes patients ask me why I have placed them on so many dangerous drugs. The answer is that the drugs collectively pose no greater danger than each alone, but the therapeutic effect of drugs in combination is startling. In this case, the whole is greater than the sum of the parts. DMARDs are any drug that reverses the actual disease process and not just the symptoms. Therefore, an antimalarial could be labeled a DMARD. The new biological response modifiers that I mention on the following pages are also DMARDs. It is just a term, but your doctor will use it, and it might confuse you unless you understand the reasons for its use.

TABLE 2

IMMUNOSUPPRESSIVE AGENTS

IMMUNOSUPPRESSIVE DRUGS*	POSITIVES	NEGATIVES
Corticosteroids (cortisone): prednisone methylprednisolone (Orazone, Medrol, Solumedrol) dexamethasone (Decadron)	Has a rapid effect on disease. Easy to ingest. Creates overall feelings of well-being and euphoria. Increases appetite. Inexpensive.	Has many side effects, such as bone loss, thinning of skin, easy bruising, sleeplessness, increased appetite, fluid retention, weight gain, cataracts.
Antimalarial: hydroxychloroquine (Plaquenil)	Gentle. Lowers cholesterol. Thins blood. Very inexpensive.	In uncoated form can cause nausea and bitter taste. May cause problems with the retina and the cornea of the eye.
Chemotherapeutics: cyclophosphamide (CytoBxan) azathioprine (Imuran) methotrexate chlorambucil (Rheumatrex)	Potent. Can reverse adverse immune reactions after oral or intravenous administration. Inexpensive.	Many side effects, including hair loss, elevated liver enzymes, suppressed bone marrow function, increased chance of infection, increased risk of cancer over the long term.

*Generic names are listed first.

Biological Response Modifiers: The Cytokine Inhibitors

You may recall that cytokines are molecules that play many roles within the immune system. One of the essential roles they play is that of messenger—that is, they promote cross-talk between the various arms of the immune system, helping to coordinate efforts to seek and destroy an antigen. The overall action of TNF is unknown, but we know that it is produced in states of profound inflammation. It serves some very important roles in the body and it can also produce many symptoms, such as weight loss and pain. For years it was believed that the ideal situation would be to find a way to interrupt the work of these cytokines.

This dream was realized in the work of Dr. Marc Feldmann and Sir Ravinder Maini of the Kennedy Institute of Rheumatology in London. In one of the most remarkable scientific quests to come along in the field of rheumatology, the two men decided to try to inhibit the TNF molecule in order to see what would happen to a patient with a chronic disease such as RA. The results of their experiments in animals and in early human studies were nothing short of miraculous and ultimately led to the formulation of the drugs *Enbrel* (etanercept), *Remicade* (infliximab), and *Humira* (adalimumab), whose sole action is to lower the levels of TNF.

The scientists found that TNF levels can be lowered in two distinct ways. First, the cytokine can be rendered inactive when bound by an antibody, which is the role of the monoclonal or very specific antibodies in the drugs Humira and Remicade, and second, it can be chemically fooled by attaching it to something that looks like its natural receptor, which blocks its effectiveness, which is the action of Enbrel. Either way, TNF is lowered and the patient, with few exceptions, improves. In September 2003, the two men won the Lasker Award for their discovery. That same year saw a newly released drug called Kineret (anakinra), that reduces the actions of the cytokine Interleukin-1β (IL-1β), which promotes inflammation in rheumatoid arthritis patients. Some RA patients have felt immeasurably better on this drug.

The concentration of TNF in the body differs with each disease. For example, this cytokine is highly elevated in rheumatoid arthritis. Therefore, lowering the levels of TNF in these patients soothes joint pain, decreases inflammation, and even halts erosion of bone, which ultimately helps keep patients free of pain. But because there is less TNF circulating in the blood of patients with diseases such as lupus and vasculitis, removal of this cytokine in these diseases does not have the same positive effect as it does in rheumatoid arthritis. To the contrary, a patient with lupus might develop new antibodies and actually get worse because of the differences in the cytokine profiles. If only for this reason, the selection of biological response modification as aform of therapy must be done with extreme care and requires a

TABLE 3

CYTOKINE INHIBITORS

CYTOKINE INHIBITOR*	POSITIVES	NEGATIVES
etanercept (Enbrel)	Inhibits TNF (tumor necrosis factor) in patients with rheumatoid arthritis. Rapidly lessens joint pain and increases mobility.	Must be injected twice weekly under the skin. Lowers resistance and allows TB or other infections, if present, to take hold. Some concern about neurological disease over long term. Very expensive.
infliximab (Remicade) adalimumab (Humira)	Inhibits TNF in patients with RA. Rapidly lessens joint pain and increases mobility.	Is administered only by IV infusion in a doctor's office or the hospital. May lead to worsening of TB and other infections. Some concern about neurological disease over long term. Very expensive.
anakinra (Kineret)	Eases symptoms in 30 to 40 percent of patients with RA.	Must be injected daily. May lead to worsening of TB and other infections. Very expensive.

*Generic names are listed first.

rheumatologist or someone with great experience in the selection of drugs and the oversight of therapy. I have to caution you that our knowledge in this area is very limited and that all people do not react equally to these biological response modifiers. The field is too new for me to make sweeping statements.

Today, rheumatoid arthritis is no longer the only disease to benefit from the cytokine inhibitors. They are currently being used very successfully in other autoimmune diseases including Crohn's disease (chronic inflammation of the bowel), uveitis (immune inflammation of the eye), and ankylosing spondylitis (a condition that causes hardening of the ligaments around the spine, with considerable pain and deformity).

Hopefully, in the future more such drugs will be released to treat an increasing number of autoimmune diseases so that even though there is no cure yet, all symptoms will be gone and the person will return to a normal life.

Additional Drugs for Treating Autoimmune Disease

▷ Cyclosporine

Cyclosporine is a very useful immunosuppressive drug that turns off cytokines so that they can no longer transmit messages. Discovered in the early 1970s, this remarkable agent immediately displayed tremendous benefits for people with transplanted organs. Before that, cortisone was the immunosuppressive drug of choice, and it had to be used in such high doses to stave off rejection that it produced extremely unpleasant side effects (see Table 2).

Cyclosporine inhibits the cytokine interleukin-2 (IL-2), which is barely detectable in diseases such as lupus and prevalent in others, such as rheumatoid arthritis. Consequently, cyclosporine is quite effective in treating rheumatoid arthritis but not necessarily in treating lupus. Unfortunately, like cortisone, cyclosporine produces many side effects in those who take it, such as high blood pressure, liver inflammation, swollen gums, and tremors. But the most serious problem with this drug is kidney disease, which can be quite dangerous. Despite these side effects, because the drug is so effective, it is still in widespread use within many autoimmune disease categories.

▷ CellCept

Mycophenolate mofetil, also known as CellCept, is FDA-approved for use to prevent rejection of transplanted organs but not officially for treating autoimmune disease. This highly potent drug targets the T and B cells. We use this drug to treat lupus and vasculitis. Side effects include nausea and bloating. Recent data suggest that CellCept can accomplish the same effect as cyclophosphamide, but with fewer side effects.

▷ Hormones

Because autoimmune diseases are so much more common to women than to men, hormone therapy for autoimmune diseases is clearly a natural direction to explore. In fact, scientists have been researching this connection for several years but have yet to come up with a potent hormone that has few side effects and will effectively counter diseases such as lupus or Sjögren's syndrome.

Several synthetic hormones are useful in treating symptoms of autoimmunity. One used to treat very low platelet counts is a weak male hormone androgen called *danocrine.* Given to patients who have low platelets—as in antiphospholipid disease or ITP—it is modestly effective, but for most other autoimmune diseases, it does very little.

A hormone that is under consideration for the treatment of lupus, which affects women ten times as often as it does men, is *dehydroepiandrosterone* (DHEA). DHEA is the most common androgen in the bodies of both men and women. It has been sold in synthetic form as a nutritional supplement in health-food stores for years. DHEA can alleviate body aches, oral ulcers, fatigue, and poor memory in some people. A problem with DHEA, and this is true for any nutritional supplement, is that because it is labeled a nutritional supplement, there is no regulation of the product, so the public has no way of knowing its maker, potency, or purity. See the following chapter for more on this subject.

Intravenous Antibodies

One form of therapy that is highly effective in the various autoimmune diseases is intravenous immunoglobulin (IVIG). This is a pooled solution of antibodies compiled from the blood of many people and then sterilized. IVIG is generally given to people who have a deficiency of antibody, but it also works in people with autoimmune disease, we think for two reasons. First, it appears to be able to block other antibodies, which slows down any immune reaction. Second, it is believed to dissolve immune complexes, which curtails inflammation, providing temporary relief from autoimmune-related symptoms. The truth is, no one really knows how it works, but we know that when it works, the results can be splendid.

IVIG is given in large doses of up to four grams per kilogram (based on the weight of the patient). The treatment is given over several hours and sometimes over several days. Patients always ask me if they can get AIDS or other diseases from IVIG, and the answer is no. Those who receive it might experience a headache or some nausea afterwards, but overall it is quite harmless. The biggest problem I see is that this drug is very expensive. In fact, most hospitals and insurance companies frown on its use because of the cost, which is approximately $3,500 per treatment. Some patients require up to two treatments a week for as long as it takes to work, which might be up to a year. Unlike most therapies, there is no fixed amount of time that constitutes a course of this particular treatment.

Bone Marrow Transplant

The use of bone marrow transplants for the treatment of autoimmune diseases is fairly new and considered somewhat risky. Bone marrow transplantation is not as complicated a procedure as it used to be, however, and it is gaining acceptance around the world. The procedure is as follows: With the patient under anesthesia, small portions of bone marrow, the breeding ground of stem cells, are removed from several sites in the patient's own body (this is called an autologous transplant) or from a genetically identical person (this is an allogenic transplant). Bone marrow may also be taken from someone who does not have the identical genetic makeup, but then the recipient's immune system has to be turned off in order to keep the donor's bone marrow from being rejected. The cells are then removed from the marrow, washed very carefully, and reserved to be reinfused intravenously into the patient. Before infusion, the patient undergoes chemotherapy or total body irradiation to disable the immune system temporarily so that it will not reject the transplanted bone marrow. The new antibody-free marrow is allowed to grow, and the patient now has a perfectly new and safe marrow.

This complicated procedure is extremely effective and lifesaving for many. Unfortunately, however, there are inherent dangers in it as well. For one, infections are common in people with suppressed immune systems. (See chapter 1 for more detail.) For another, there is a condition called graft-versus-host (GVH) disease (discussed in chapter 15 on scleroderma), in which the body rejects tissue that comes from another human being who differs in some genetic way. This can cause life-threatening complications. For these reasons, bone marrow transplants are given only to patients who are the most ill and cannot be satisfactorily treated well with conventional drugs. It is essential for patients to investigate this procedure well and pursue it with only the most experienced physicians.

Progress on the Treatment Front

A large number of drugs are on the horizon for people with autoimmune diseases, making this a most exciting time for physician and patient alike. Unlike the current drugs we have discussed above, these drugs attack specific parts of cells. Here are some of the newest of the new:

> ▷ *Rituximab.* A biological response modifier, Rituximab binds to a receptor on the B cell called CD20. Originally used for various forms of blood cancer, this agent may be quite effective in treating rheumatoid arthritis and lupus. RA was once considered an illness of the T cells, but we now know that B cells are just as involved in this disease. In the case of lupus,

we have known for a long time that B cells are responsible for antibody production and other aspects of this illness. This drug targets certain markers on B cells and kills them, allowing new B cells to grow that do not have the disease properties of the old cells.

▷ *CTLA4Ig* Another new drug for rheumatoid arthritis, CTLA4Ig is so new that it does not yet have a name. This drug blocks the immune response by attacking *costimulatory molecules* on cells. A costimulatory molecule is one that has to be tweaked (forgive the nonscientific vernacular, but I can think of no better word) before an actual cell function will follow. In other words, you can prevent an immune reaction if you disrupt certain aspects of the workings of the cell, which is what CTLA4Ig is designed to do.

▷ *SCIO 469.* Before an enzyme becomes a cytokine, SCIO 469 attacks it, so, essentially, an immune reaction is inhibited. This design has great promise for diseases such as RA, but it has no current use for any other disease.

▷ Three more drugs are in development for the treatment of lupus and antiphospholipid syndrome. One drug, specific for lupus, includes agents that deal with *tolerance*, that is, the immune system's ability to accept certain antigens and not respond to them. The principle behind this drug is as follows: If a person could be made tolerant against an antigen, the immune system might bypass the antigen as "self" and not attack it. Two other drugs, one for lupus-related kidney disease and one for antiphospholipid syndrome, use this principle of *tolerization*. These drugs are so new they have not yet been named.

Many of you are no doubt awed, as I am, by the panoply of new drugs used to treat various diseases, but others will ask "Why don't I see any help for scleroderma or newer agents for lupus?" If you are wondering why rheumatoid arthritis has so much new therapy and diseases like scleroderma and multiple sclerosis do not, I will do my best to explain. Diseases like scleroderma are very complex and not yet understood well enough to easily develop new agents that would reverse the illness. They affect far fewer people than RA. While the true causes of diseases such as RA are also not clear, they affect millions more people than scleroderma and are therefore bigger targets for the pharmaceutical world. I have not excluded any new drugs for the so-called "orphan" diseases in this book; it is just that there are few.

One of my goals in writing this book is to prompt legislators and powerful people who are affected in some way by these autoimmune conditions to understand the complexities of the disease and the impact that even the rarest of illnesses has on the quality of millions of lives. It is essential that they know, as we doctors do, that these diseases strike people from all paths of life, many of whom are without means and must rely on the achievements of a few smart scientists and the financial decisions and directions of our leaders in Congress, particularly those who control the directions of the pharmaceutical industry. Some of my patients have told me that polio was cured because President Franklin Roosevelt had it, implying that the only way attention will be drawn to the autoimmune diseases is if someone of prominence is stricken. I, of course, believe there is already far too much autoimmune disease in this world, and for my part, I am attempting to garner the same attention within these pages for the 22 million women who have these illnesses, but who lack a voice.

Living Well

While living well is not exactly a drug per se, I include it in this chapter because I believe caring for yourself is every bit as important as other types of therapy. It is a wonderful gift that only you can give to yourself. Believe it or not, one of the best treatments for immune disorders is bed rest. I know, try telling that to someone with a type A personality, which sometimes seems to describe around 99 percent of our society. (That statistic is a guess, incidentally, but I formulate it on my patient base, and, I admit it, on myself.) That the immune system responds to rest is a given. It also responds well to a balanced diet, healthy activity, exercising, and getting enough sleep—all of which I mention in chapter 1. Right up there in importance, though, is maintaining a positive frame of mind.

I have said this earlier but it bears repeating: The right attitude is key to living well with autoimmune diseases, perhaps more so than in any other diseases I have come across in my many years in practice. As I note in chapter 20, I strongly believe in a mind-body connection, and that connection is largely the work of the immune system. There is much scientific data to support the notion that a healthy attitude will benefit a patient by helping traditional medicine work well. That is not to say you can read a few funny comic books and, poof! you are cured. But such an attitude helps the drugs prescribed work at peak efficiency. How this works, no one really knows, but studies tell us that frequent laughter has been shown to improve immune function, raise resistance to infection, and increase life span. Is it easy to always be in a positive frame of mind in the face of a disease for which there is no known cause or cure? Of course not. But it is my job to tell you all I know, and I know that attitude truly counts. Perhaps this is why most of the comedians I have known, and some I have had as patients, live so long and with such a great quality of life.

CHAPTER TWENTY

ALTERNATIVE AND COMPLEMENTARY THERAPIES

> ## From Acupuncture to Zinc

HE TERM *ALTERNATIVE medicine* refers to certain techniques that patients sometimes substitute for allopathic (conventional) medical care. *Complementary medicine*, on the other hand, refers to noninvasive, nonpharmaceutical techniques used as a complement to conventional medical treatments, such as drugs and surgery. In this case, conventional medicine is the primary tool and the noninvasive, nonpharmaceutical techniques are used as a supplement.

Alternative and complementary therapies are becoming more widely known and available to everyone. For some people, looking outside of mainstream conventional medicine provides a feeling of being able to take some control in an otherwise uncontrollable situation. The popularity of these therapies continues to soar. In 1993, a study in the *New England Journal of Medicine* stated that one of three people in this country used some kind of alternative (or complementary) medicine in the previous year. Newer studies show the numbers growing exponentially. In response, the National Institutes of Health added a federal agency in 1998 called the National Center for

Complementary and Alternative Medicine (NCCAM). Additionally, at least two-thirds of medical schools in the United States now offer courses in complementary and alternative medicine (CAM).

I must admit that early on I was very skeptical of any complementary and alternative treatments. But I now see the value inherent in many of the complementary ones. On the other hand, I do *not* agree with the use of alternative treatments for autoimmune diseases. Substituting a questionable therapy—that is, one which has not been scientifically proven—for a treatment that we know can keep you alive, or at the very least keep symptoms at bay, reminds me of the days when people searching for a cancer cure curtailed their medical treatment and flew to Mexico to be cured by a serum made from avocado pits. I still do not understand it.

While scientific evidence exists to confirm the safety and efficacy of some complementary therapies, most remain untested, and if they have been tested, sometimes the methods of testing have been less than scientific. Many so-called natural remedies seem harmless and do not come with a daunting list of adverse effects, but that is only because they are not required by law in this country to do so. Some are not harmless and can, in fact, cause injury or death to patients who have taken them. If an herb is not FDA sanctioned, then who knows for sure if it is truly natural, and who, exactly, is there to say what is and is not a remedy? If you have a piece of paper and some glue, you have a label. If you have a printer, you can make that label say anything you want it to. Just keep this in mind: When it comes to some of these miracle potions, nobody is watching anybody.

Lest you think that I am against complementary treatments altogether, let me set the record straight. Many of these treatments do work to make people feel better. I have the word of a great many patients on that, and I always trust what my patients tell me.

On the following pages, I provide a brief overview of some of the more common alternative and complementary therapies. The treatments include drugs, nutritional supplements, and other therapies. I have included both alternative and complementary regimens, although I have not labeled them as such because I do not know how people use them. Some patients may exchange any of these for existing treatment while others just add them to their existing treatment plan. As you will see, I sanction some of these methods and am opposed to others, which I include because they have become so popular that they merit discussion. On some, the jury is still out. The information you will read here comes from my patients, colleagues, and, where available, the medical literature. Hopefully, new data from ongoing studies will be available in the next few years and will shed more light on this constantly evolving area.

A caveat: Before employing *any* of these methods, it is essential to discuss them with your personal physician. If you seek more information about these modalities, you can find help in the suggested reading or list of helpful organizations in the appendices.

▷ *Acupuncture*

The Chinese therapy of acupuncture—a procedure that involves the placement of fine needles into specific areas of the body—has been around for millennia and is an increasingly popular treatment for pain. Science does not fully understand the mechanisms by which this modality works, but the results are quite real. Scans show that the metabolism of the brain changes during an acupuncture treatment. It is apparent as well that the procedures have some real effects on blood flow and possibly even on the immune system. Endorphins (natural pain-relieving molecules) and hormones also are likely released when the needles are placed. Done correctly, acupuncture cannot cause harm, and I often recommend it for patients in severe pain. In China, it is routinely and successfully used during surgery to augment the effects of standard anesthetics. Many of my patients with myositis and fibromyalgia use acupuncture and are happy with the results.

The FDA now regulates acupuncture needles and tools with the same standards they use for surgical instruments, but it is up to you to find a licensed acupuncture practitioner. Because more and more physicians are becoming aware of this particular therapy, your physician may be able to recommend someone. In fact, many medical doctors, including neurologists, anesthesiologists, and specialists in physical medicine, are themselves becoming trained acupuncturists. Today, many states have established training standards for certification in acupuncture, but the requirements for licensure vary. Be aware, too, that while certification indicates that the practitioner has met certain standards to treat patients with acupuncture, credentials do not always ensure competency. Many things can go wrong with acupuncture. One can place the needle in the wrong place, transmit infections such as hepatitis C, and produce a huge bruise if a blood vessel is struck. My personal concern about tattooists and acupuncture specialists, although it may be unfair to lump them together, is infection. The real acupuncturists take great care to maintain sterile instruments.

▷ *Ayurveda and Holistic Medicine*

Ayurveda comes from two Sanskrit root words: *ayus*, meaning life and *veda*, meaning knowledge or science. This nontraditional medicine began in India, where it has been in use for thousands of years, but it is becoming well known and accepted in the West now as well. The principles are centered on rejuvenation and are based on the integration of spiritual, mental, and physical balance. Ayurveda is similar to holistic medicine, which emphasizes treating the whole person, not just the illness. Both of these methods include diet restrictions, exercise, and a steady routine of nutritional supplements and herbs to be used for disease prevention and treatment. I cannot say this often enough: Be aware that any herbs used as part of this or other treatments are not regulated, and our knowledge of what most herbs do to the immune system is not known. Some of my patients swear by these two philosophies. If it works for you, great. But remember, this form of medicine can safely be used only in conjunction with conventional medicine. It should not be a substitute for it.

▷ *Cetyl Myristoleate (CMO)*

This is a waxy fatty acid that is sometimes touted in the tabloids as a cure for arthritis. I do not recommend it, because no data that I know of describes CMO's effects on humans. Many years ago a strain of mice with an artificial form of arthritis got better when given this fatty acid. That is all I know of it, other than that the chemical is very expensive and the manufacturer prefers that the person taking this go off any and all other chemotherapeutic agents. That in itself raises a red flag for me. *In no case should any drugs for autoimmune disease be stopped without the sanction of the treating physician.* The results can be tragic. My advice? Stay away from CMO.

▷ Chiropractic Manipulation

I believe that there is a very welcome place for chiropractic manipulation in the treatment of autoimmune-associated diseases, particularly chronic-pain-associated diseases such as fibromyalgia. Both high-velocity and low-velocity adjustments by a chiropractor have found a place in the treatment of the chronic pain. The benefits may include pain relief and muscle relaxation.

▷ Copper and Zinc

The theory that copper has a positive effect on arthritis goes back to the ancient Egyptians. Copper is a metal that supports certain enzymes in the body. Enzymes help in digestion and promote biochemical reactions in the body, some of which are essential to good health. For example, certain enzymes neutralize the effects of free radicals—atoms that are formed when oxygen interacts with certain molecules. Once formed, these highly reactive radicals can start a chain reaction, eventually damaging the cells and causing inflammation. To prevent free radical damage, the body has a defense system of *antioxidants*—molecules that interact with free radicals and cancel the chain reaction before damage is done. Enzymes in the body boost these antioxidants; and copper supports the enzymes, thus preventing cellular damage and, ultimately, inflammation.

Zinc is another essential mineral that is found in almost every cell. Like copper, zinc supports a healthy immune system. In addition, it is needed for wound healing and DNA synthesis, and helps the body grow and develop as it should. Zinc is found in a wide variety of foods, including oysters, red meat, and poultry. Beans, nuts, dairy products, and whole grains are other sources of zinc. Supplements are also available in pill form.

Because copper and zinc act as antioxidants, taking both of those minerals, particularly for people with joint problems associated with rheumatoid arthritis, is beneficial, and taking the two minerals together helps maintain a proper balance.

Here are two questions I am asked at least once a month by patients with rheumatoid arthritis: Do copper bracelets work? Should I purchase a zinc necklace? I tell them, if you think you look good in copper and zinc, why not? But wearing this metallic jewelry for the purposes of alleviating symptoms, I'm not so sure. To date, I have not read a convincing report that they work.

▷ *Diet and Nutritional Regimens*

A well-balanced diet is an integral component of any treatment program. Along with exercise, healthy eating helps with body weight. This is no small matter for people with certain autoimmune diseases, particularly multiple sclerosis and rheumatoid arthritis, because extra weight puts extra pressure on joints and muscles. For many years, the use of diet to treat diseases of the immune system was thought to be a form of quackery. For example, in a 1981 book entitled *The Truth About Diet and Arthritis*, the Arthritis Foundation reported, "The simple proven fact is, no food has anything to do with causing arthritis, and no food is effective in treating or curing it."

Today, we know better. There is considerable information about using food to enhance immune function, although controversy among experts still exists. Because this is such a big topic, I cannot begin to cover thoroughly the data on nutrition for people with autoimmune diseases. Instead, I suggest that you explore some of the many books and government pamphlets that are available on the topics of particular interest to you. I do, however, want to mention two food-connected issues that I know to be helpful for women with autoimmune diseases:

▷ As an irrepressibly devoted fan of sushi, I was encouraged to learn that cold-water fish contain a substance called *eicosapentanoic acid* (EPA) that is incorporated in our cells. EPA is one of several omega-3 fatty acids used by the body to synthesize the chemicals that cause inflammation. In this way, the omega-3 fatty acids have been shown to modify, although we do not know to what degree, the immune response and may be helpful in treating inflammatory autoimmune diseases such as rheumatoid arthritis, arthritis connected to psoriasis, Raynaud's phenomenon, MS, and lupus. Foods that have EPA-like substances in them include dairy products, organ meats, and flaxseed. Although our main dietary sources of EPA are cold-water fish, fish oil supplements also may raise the body's EPA concentrations. If you intend to purchase EPA as a dietary supplement, I suggest you check with your retailer for the most reputable manufacturer. As with all other food supplements, the quality of EPA may vary.

▷ Nutrition researchers have shown that the consumption of certain vegetables appears to be helpful in the treatment of autoimmune diseases. A few studies demonstrate that eating a diet high in cruciferate vegetables—including broccoli, brussels sprouts, cabbage, and kale—or taking capsules of the extract of these vegetables can mitigate estrogen metabolism in women. As estrogens tend to boost the immune system, it is believed that diminishing estrogen will help ameliorate those diseases directly affected by estrogens. The disease that is most clearly affected by estrogen is lupus. However, there are data to show that multiple sclerosis and rheumatoid arthritis are affected as well. One study showed that women who were pure vegetarians for some time had less strong menstrual periods, tended to be calmer, and had less of a risk for breast and possibly ovarian cancer. The jury is out on this, since only a few studies have yet been published. However, this kind of dietary insight offers fascinating possibilities for the future.

While we are on the subject of diet, I want to mention dietary or nutritional supplements, which are often reported by patients as helpful in treating rheumatic diseases. These include products such as S-adenosylmethionine (SAM-e) for osteoarthritis and fibromyalgia, dehydroepiandrosterone (DHEA) for lupus, and glucosamine and chondroitin sulfate for osteoarthritis, all of which are discussed in this chapter. Although these supplements are considered by the U.S. Food and Drug Administration (FDA) as foods, they are regulated differently from other foods and from drugs. Most often, classification as a dietary supplement is determined by the information that the manufacturer provides on the product label or in accompanying literature, although many food and dietary supplement product labels do not include this information. The label of a dietary supplement may even describe how the product affects certain body organs or systems, but they cannot mention any specific disease. An example of such a statement, which does not require FDA approval, might be that the product helps you relax. The message here is to look beyond a label before you take any dietary supplements. Check first with your doctor, because some of these can counteract the medicines you are currently taking.

▷ *Exercise and Rest*

Exercise is essential for good health and for most people with autoimmune disease. Physical exercise can reduce joint pain and stiffness and increase flexibility, muscle strength, and endurance. It also helps with weight reduction and contributes to an improved sense of well-being. In short: The immune system responds well to exercise, and everyone who can exercise should do so. But pay close attention to signals from your body. Understand that if you experience pain or fatigue, you must take a break and rest. On the other hand, too much rest may cause muscles and joints to become stiff. There are three types of exercise to consider:

> ▷ Range-of-motion exercises, such as stretching, help keep joints moving normally, increase flexibility, and relieve stiffness.
> ▷ Strengthening exercises, such as lifting weights, keep muscles strong. Strong muscles help support and protect joints affected by arthritis.
> ▷ Aerobic exercises, such as walking, running, biking, and swimming, improve cardiovascular fitness and help control weight. Done in moderation, aerobic exercise is particularly good for people with fibromyalgia and multiple sclerosis.

People with diseases such as polymyositis and dermatomyositis, in which the muscles are inflamed, should be alert to exercises that can overstress muscle, such as isometrics. The best advice I can offer is that you develop a comfortable balance between rest and activity. *Before starting any exercise program, talk with your doctor.*

▷ *Ginger*

Ginger root is a staple of many diets, particularly in the Far East. Ayurvedic healing systems in India prescribe the use of ginger as an antidote to inflammation. Ginger supplements, which are available in various forms, probably work on inflammation by inhibiting prostaglandins and leukotrienes (inflammatory chemicals), but there is no available human data that I know of to support the claim. One study I read advised that rats with joint inflammation did well on ginger for about a month. (I am only reporting this; I am not supporting it.)

▷ *Glucosamine and Chondroitin*

Glucosamine and chondroitin are proteins found in and around our bodies' cartilage cells. Without this smooth and springy substance, the bones scrape against each other, causing chronic pain and limiting range of motion. Symptoms of rheumatoid arthritis can result from a breakdown of cartilage. Glucosamine inhibits inflammation and stimulates cartilage cell growth, while chondroitin provides cartilage with strength and resilience. Researchers believe taking these substances in the form of food supplements may help in the repair and maintenance of natural cartilage. I also believe that these agents work. Although this is used more commonly for people with osteoarthritis, I have interviewed many patients with rheumatoid arthritis who say it makes them feel better, and I have talked to researchers in Boston and in the Netherlands who have published data on this supplement's efficacy.

A warning: *Patients who are taking the blood-thinning medication heparin—which has molecular structure similar to chondroitin—should have their blood-clotting activity monitored if they add chondroitin to their diets, because taking both at the same time could increase the risk of bleeding.*

If you choose to take these dietary supplements, you should be aware that they are not cheap. A month's supply of glucosamine (at 1,500 milligrams a day, the amount used in most studies) can run from thirty to sixty dollars. Researchers at the University of Maryland School of Pharmacy in Baltimore recently tested several brands and found greatly varying amounts of glucosamine and chondroitin in each, and sometimes not as much as their labels indicated. While I cannot suggest a specific brand, I do suggest you find an experienced person in a reputable health-food store or drugstore and discuss your choice before purchasing.

▷ *Gold*

Gold has had truly amazing effects on autoimmune disease. It has been prescribed as a nonalternative drug for years, particularly for rheumatoid arthritis. Gold acts in a way that no one has been able to precisely explain, nor can we say exactly how it affects the body, but there is much data to show that it really does work. Gold inhibits bacterial growth in the test tube, and some actually believe that it inhibits the growth of the organisms that cause arthritis, even though no organisms have been identified as the cause of that condition. More detailed information on gold and how it is administered can be found on page 199 in chapter 17, Rheumatoid Arthritis.

▷ *Herbal Supplements*

An herb (also called a botanical) is a plant or plant part used for its scent, flavor, and/or therapeutic properties. Although many herbs have a long history of use and of claimed health benefits, I strongly disagree with the use of herbal supplements in treating autoimmune disease. Here is why:

▷ Most herbal preparations stimulate immune function, and that is in direct opposition to our therapeutic goal for autoimmune diseases.

▷ Any herb that is used for medicinal purposes should be analyzed, the active ingredients isolated, and the pure materials tested first in animals for safety and then in humans. But the government does not regulate them, and so herbs can contain unknown substances. Identifying the active ingredients in herbs and understanding how herbs affect the body are important research areas for the National Center for Complementary and Alternative Medicine.

▷ Toxic impurities and incorrectly mixed herbs can result in kidney failure or death. (I read a study recently in which a young woman with lupus suffered from renal [kidney] failure from taking an herb called "cat's claw.")

▷ Some herbal supplements can counteract the effects of the immunosuppressive drugs that are given to control illness.

▷ Many so-called "natural" or "herbal" tablets (usually sold to patients on the black market in this country or in various guises in foreign countries) contain anti-inflammatory drugs, cortisone-like steroids, and even amphetamine stimulants within them (see chapter 4 on ITP). These can temporarily induce good feelings and relieve pain but may also mask the true problem, which might be getting worse.

▷ The interaction of some of these mysterious agents on concurrent medications taken to affect the immune system is unknown. Patients on antiseizure medicine who take evening primrose oil, for example, can actually increase their potential for seizure.

Research may someday find a place for herbs in the treatment of connective tissue diseases, but until they have been standardized, as prescription drugs are, they are best avoided. Once more, with feeling: *No one should ever use an herbal supplement after a diagnosis of an autoimmune disease.*

▷ *Homeopathy*

This form of medicine bases its conclusions on the life force. I must admit that when a patient tells me this about homeopathy, it makes me think of *Star Wars*. Homeopathy, I'm sorry to say, is not likely to make your immune system better or cure autoimmune diseases. Just as I am generally against the use of herbs, for reasons I mention above, so too am I against homeopathy as a treatment for autoimmune disease. The reasons are similar. The last thing an overactive immune system needs is something to stimulate it even more.

The principle of homeopathy is to take a natural substance that produces specific symptoms, such as diarrhea in a healthy person, and give it to a sick person in diluted form. When I was a student, we referred to homeopathy as a means of making you better by making you sick. Most of the time the herbal material is so diluted in solution as to be completely ineffective, but I still do not like the idea of something not approved by the FDA being used to treat disease, any disease. Besides, numerous published studies have shown no benefit to homeopathy in the arthritic diseases, and no specific mention is made of any efficacy in the treatment of immune disorders.

▷ Hormones

The only alternative or complementary medicine that that I know of that is also a hormone is DHEA (dehyroepiandrosterone). Fortunately, DHEA may soon become a legitimate therapy for patients with mild to moderate lupus. Clinical trials are over, and they have shown the drug to have beneficial effects for lupus and perhaps some other diseases, such as osteoporosis. We are awaiting final approval from the FDA for this agent. Other than mild acne, DHEA has very few side effects. People feel better, have a stronger sex drive, and reportedly have better memory. At this time I would suggest people who suffer from autoimmune diseases, particularly those with attendant weakness and fatigue, should discuss taking DHEA with their physicians. It may help. There is more discussion of DHEA in chapters 10, 12, and 19.

▷ Magnets and Electromagnetic Fields

Patients with arthritic and autoimmune diseases generally use static magnets (the ones you fasten to your body) to get rid of pain and inflammation. I am sorry to report that there is very little data to support the use of static magnets in any kind of autoimmune or arthritic disease. There are many uncontrolled observations and personal testimonials to their use, but as a scientist, the only research I can subscribe to is controlled, in which people are placed randomly into treatment or nontreatment groups, and after a period of time the results for each group are compared for specific parameters, such as pain relief or ease of movement. As far as I am aware, the efficacy of magnets for autoimmune diseases has never been proven by a controlled study.

▷ *Massage Therapy*

Having someone massage your sore and painful muscles and joints is one of life's great gifts. You do need to tell the masseuse or masseur that you are ill, however, and tell them the kind of pressure that works for you. Most competent and certified massage therapists know how to care for patients with certain diseases. Increase of blood flow to the affected areas and the overall well-being that this form of therapy produces can be very relaxing and rewarding for those who can afford it. I always offer a note of caution for fibromyalgia patients: Make sure that that your rheumatologist sanctions your plan and that you take an analgesic directly afterward to prevent possible pain.

▷ *Methyl Sulfonyl Methane (MSM)*

Methyl sulfonyl methane (MSM) is a derivative of *dimethyl sulfoxide* (DMSO), which has been in use for years, although perhaps not as commonly now as in the past few decades. MSM is an organic sulfur compound that smells like raw clams. I can recall in my days at Rockefeller when the entire clinic area smelled like the ocean on a bad day, after certain physicians would swab large amounts of DMSO on a patient's swollen joints. Most of the anecdotal reports of the effects of this compound come from patients who took the drug in pill form for osteoarthritis, which is not an autoimmune disease. However, there are reports of swollen salivary glands improving with application of MSM in liquid form. I also have heard stories about the healing of ulcers on scleroderma-affected hands, and of the relief of joint pains with rheumatoid arthritis. Because there have been no controlled trials using this drug, I would caution interested patients who intend to use the agent that, despite the many anecdotal accolades, there is nothing proven about MSM's use in the autoimmune diseases. Talk with your physician before considering MSM.

▷ *Melatonin*

Melatonin is a hormone that regulates the biological clock. For this reason, young doctors on call trying to get sleep at off hours and airline pilots who want to overcome jet lag ingest this drug. Many people think of melatonin as a sleeping aid, and some patients have requested it to help them sleep. I explain that melatonin may actually increase immune activity, so *it should be considered off-limits by anyone with an autoimmune disease.*

▷ *Mind-Body Therapies*

For my money, mind-body therapies are among the most promising areas of treatment of the immune diseases. Mind-body therapies have been shown to increase quality of life, reduce pain, and improve symptoms for people with chronic diseases and health conditions. They may also help control and reverse certain diseases, particularly those that are stress-related. They pose little risk, are generally inexpensive, and most have few side effects. The rigorous data produced by a number of investigators shows a direct relationship between the mind and the immune system. Many of my patients swear by these methods.

Many techniques draw upon the connections between the mind and the body. These include meditation, mindfulness training, biofeedback, prayer, and faith healing. Progressive relaxation and yoga are other common methods used to relieve stress and they are also useful in the management of the chronic autoimmune diseases. Moreover, if, as we believe, the immune system follows the brain's commands, it is likely that stress relief will have a good and lasting effect on the overall disease.

Meditation. The goal of meditation is to calm and focus the mind. When performed on a regular basis, meditation is an efficient way of promoting relaxation. This discipline involves two basic components: (1) repetitive focus on a word, sound, prayer, phrase, body sensation, or muscular activity and (2) the adoption of a passive attitude toward intruding thoughts and a return to the focus.

Mindfulness training. Awareness of the present moment is the essential discipline on mindfulness training. Lack of awareness and attention can lead to stress and bad health habits. To be mindful is to participate fully in whatever one is doing at the present moment, whether reading, walking, working, eating, exercising, relaxing, and so on.

Biofeedback. Special instruments that measure and display heart rate, perspiration, muscle tension, and other indicators of stress and physiological activity are used in biofeedback. Patients can observe their measurements and learn to consciously control functions that were previously unconsciously controlled.

Prayer and faith healing and *yoga* are two more mind-body techniques that are discussed elsewhere in this chapter.

Costs can vary widely for mind-body treatments, depending on the type and the kind of training of the practitioner. Many insurance companies will reimburse some mind-body treatments and training sessions. Consumers should be aware of their insurance provisions.

▷ *Oral Collagen*

A few small studies suggest that oral type II chicken collagen may be beneficial to some with rheumatoid arthritis, acting by a process known as oral tolerance. I like to think of oral tolerance as immune obfuscation. The immune system becomes overloaded with antigens and does not act because of overexposure. (We also give intravenous drugs to produce tolerance, and it is very effective. This method can act as "desensitization for diseases such as lupus, RA, and MS.) There is currently a large multicenter trial going on to prove the efficacy of collagen for RA.

Collagen can be derived from shark cartilage as well as chicken, but the advantageous results come only from chicken collagen, so be sure to read labels carefully. Chicken collagen is available as capsules and tablets, but because of lack of longterm safety studies, nutritional supplements containing chicken collagen should be avoided by pregnant women and nursing mothers. Those with rheumatoid arthritis who are interested in trying chicken collagen should consult with their physicians before doing so.

▷ *Religion and Spiritual Beliefs*

Bringing religion and prayer into the treatment arena may be controversial, but it works for many people. According to a Johns Hopkins study, people who are more spiritual are better able to deal with the discomforts and limitations of chronic disease than those who are less spiritual. For the purposes of the study, spirituality was defined as "the capacity of an individual to stand outside of his or her immediate sense of time and place and to view life from a larger, more detached perspective." The study involved seventy-seven patients over age thirty who had had rheumatoid arthritis for at least two years. The conclusion showed that while being spiritual did not reduce the effects of the arthritis, reduce pain, or improve mobility, the more spiritual people were happier and felt better about their health overall.

I once had a patient who never went into a hospital that did not have a religious connection. For example, he would go only to Mount Sinai, Our Lady of Perpetual something, or Saint this or that. He swore that he could be healed only in such an environment. I believe the stress relief that religion brings to an individual—the organized relaxation, the inner calm, and the alteration of life's bad habits toward good ones (stop smoking, decrease drinking, get closer to family, and so on) is likely to have beneficial effects on the overall person and ultimately on the immune system. I like to think of religion as being similar to psychiatric help in time of need. The effects on the immune system must be quantified at some point, but I do not see a grant being funded for this purpose in the near future. (Although I have a feeling that many novenas have been said in hopes that it would.)

▷ *Shark Cartilage*

There is no good evidence that the cartilage of a shark, which can be taken in both pill and powder form, has any effect on the autoimmune diseases. It has been used for patients with discoid lupus—a skin disorder that affects the face, scalp, and other areas of the body (see chapter 10)—and rheumatoid arthritis, but without much success. Studies of this agent show that it helps grow blood vessels in the test tube and that it inhibits tumor cell growth. I include it here only because this has had such a popular run in the tabloids that I believe its influence, or noninfluence, on these diseases should be noted. On the other hand, oral collagen from chickens (see page 87) has had more promising results.

▷ Spa and Balneotherapy

We all know what a spa is, but I have only recently learned about balneotherapy, which describes bathing in mineral waters. Mineral baths have been around for hundreds of years and have been frequented by popes, kings, queens, and all variety of glitterati. While this therapy is no replacement for the standard therapy for chronic illnesses, it plays a lovely complementary role, and there are no adverse effects. I have been in a variety of mineral pools, both heated and unheated, from Iceland to Israel, and find them to be very relaxing. People with joint pain and chronic pain conditions are said to improve with this kind of treatment. The effects of balneotherapy on the immune system await better research, and I, for one, am ready to volunteer as a principal investigator for the study!

I will share one scenario that is likely to get me into hot water. At a recent International Phospholipid meeting in Sapporo, Japan, the guidelines for the diagnosis of the "sticky blood syndrome" were established. All of the immunologists, hematologists, rheumatologists, and a smattering of orthopedists went to a volcanic spa in the mountains for balneotherapy. I do not believe that it did anything for our knowledge of the antiphospholipid syndrome, but it relaxed all of us, save one, who had to be resuscitated for drinking too much sake after his bath.

▷ Venoms

Just the idea of snake, ant, and bee venoms gives me the creeps. I admit it. But it is true that some of these venoms are considered to be therapies for the immune disorders. Early in the 1960s, for example, one investigator found that snake venom prevented overall inflammation. Given to rabbits, snake venom also decreased the formation of immune complexes. However, most of the studies of rats and mice treated with cobra venom and that of some other serpents showed no long-lasting improvement of their conditions. To my knowledge, ant venom trials have not been scientifically conducted, but there is one inconclusive study using ant venom in the treatment of rheumatoid arthritis in which the investigators claim some degree of symptomatic relief for their patients after two weeks of therapy.

Bee venom treatment includes *apitherapy,* which uses bee products to promote healing, and *apipuncture,* which employs bee stings for the same purpose. These therapies for immune and arthritic diseases have been around since ancient times. A recent article in the *New York Times Magazine* indicated that bee stings have a remitting effect on the symptoms of multiple sclerosis. While it is true that certain parts of the bee's venom can produce anti-inflammatory effects, most experts believe that you would require so much bee venom to get a significant response that you would surely suffer first from other nonintended effects. Personally, I do not believe there is any benefit to being stung by bees or taking injections of bee venom under the skin.

▷ Yoga

I am all for yoga. I have seen no studies that scientifically evaluate the effects of yoga to control symptoms of the autoimmune diseases, but I do have anecdotal evidence from my patients. They rave about yoga and its ability to manage pain, high blood pressure, diabetes, and depression. They say the stretching and the relaxation and the mental discipline are all helpful.

According to the American Yoga Association, yoga helps many people with arthritis deal with pain and stiffness, improve range of motion, and increase strength for daily activities. A pilot study published in the *British Journal of Rheumatology* states that the benefits of low-impact exercises such as yoga may extend to people with rheumatoid arthritis. Yoga poses including range-of-motion, muscle strengthening, and endurance exercises—the three major forms of exercise typically prescribed for people with RA.

Some Controversial Alternative and Complementary Treatments

Even though the following appear to be standard medical treatments, they are used—if they *are* used—alongside other more scientific regimens, which is why I have included them here. I find them both to be highly controversial methods of treating autoimmune disease, but some doctors still find them useful. (Accordingly, you will see a discussion on apheresis in the chapter on PANDAS.)

▷ Antibiotics

Antibiotics are tried and true methods of combating some types of infection. The only antibiotic that I can say really works for the autoimmune diseases is *minocycline,* which is part of the tetracycline family. This drug is considered an unorthodox method of treating certain autoimmune diseases and, indeed, there is much controversy over its use, but the data are very positive for some groups of patients. Published data show minocycline, an antibiotic, provides symptomatic improvement in some patients with rheumatoid arthritis. For other diseases, I suggest caution, because minocycline has been associated with the development of drug-induced lupus.

▷ Apheresis

In the 1970s, before we had many of the drugs we now have, removing the source of toxic self-reacting cells—that is, antibodies—from the blood was the method of choice for certain autoimmune diseases. In this procedure, large amounts of plasma and cells (generally three units of the total six that are in the body) are drawn intravenously from the patient and spun down in a centrifuge to remove the plasma. The blood is then run through a machine where it is cleaned of antibodies, and then intravenously reinfused back into the patient. The procedure initially makes a patient "plasma poor," but with the addition of a saline solution, the blood volume quickly returns. Two diseases, lupus and RA, were of particular interest to investigators in those days, but the plan was for all of the autoimmune disorders to eventually be treated in this way. In the case of lupus, the idea was to rid the blood of antibody in order to prevent organ damage resulting from immune complexes. In rheumatoid arthritis, the goal was to achieve a remission.

Removing autoantibodies by apheresis (which is sometimes called plasmapheresis) is a good idea, but from my experience, it rarely works in patients with lupus. It is sometimes used in PANDAS (see chapter 7) with moderate success, but in the end, new and higher amounts of antibodies can return, so sometimes patients can get worse. In Germany, apheresis is combined with chemotherapy to treat lupus-related kidney disease with reportedly positive effects.

Another process, similar to apheresis, involves removing plasma and passing it over a glass column that has been filled with an absorbing substance. The substance removes certain inflammatory molecules (cytokines) from the blood before the blood is passed back into the patient's arm. This procedure is approved only for rheumatoid arthritis, however, because among the cytokines it removes are TNF and certain others which are directly associated with that particular disease.

GLOSSARY

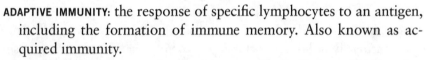

ADAPTIVE IMMUNITY: the response of specific lymphocytes to an antigen, including the formation of immune memory. Also known as acquired immunity.

ALKALINE PHOSPHATASE: a chemical present in the liver and bones that can be found in high concentration in patients with primary billiary cirrhosis.

ALOPECIA AREATA UNIVERSALIS: an autoimmune disease that causes loss of all hair on the head and body.

ANALGESIC: a medication that relieves pain by blocking pain receptors.

ANDROGENS: male hormones.

ANTIBODY: a protein in the blood that binds to a specific target called an antigen, resulting in an immune complex.

ANTIGEN: a foreign molecule that enters the body and triggers an immune reaction.

ANTIGEN PRESENTATION: the offering of a substance to a cell—such as a fragment of protein or a fat or a sugar—that processes it for the immune system. The T and B cells learn about antigens in this way.

ANTIGEN PRESENTING CELLS: macrophages, B cells, and dendritic cells that process antigens and display the fragments of the antigen on the surface of a cell, allowing the T cells come to recognize the antigen.

ANTIPHOSPHOLIPID SYNDROME: a condition characterized by antibodies to fat proteins on cells. Usually associated with sticky blood, strokes, or blood clots.

Glossary

ANTISTREPTOLYSIN TEST: a test in which antibodies are measured against the chemical that comes out of a bacterium known as the strepto-coccus. Used in diagnosing rheumatic fever.

ANTITOXIN: an antibody directed against a poison, or an antigen, that is injected into a person to provide rapid immunity.

APOPTOSIS: programmed cell death. Every cell in the human body is programmed to die at a certain time.

AUTOANTIBODY: manufactured by the immune system in response to a perceived antigen.

AUTOANTIGEN: molecules that exist naturally within the body but for some unknown reason are perceived as foreign by the immune system.

AUTOIMMUNE RESPONSE: the immune system's response to an autoantigen.

AUTOREACTIVITY: another term for an autoimmune response involving both antibodies and lymphocytes.

AZATHIOPRINE: a potent immunosuppressive drug that kills rapidly pro-liferating lymphocytes, thereby slowing the immune response. Used to treat autoimmune muscle diseases, rheumatoid arthritis, lupus, and others.

B LYMPHOCYTE: one of the two major kinds of lymphocytes that can re-act with antigen. Matures to make a plasma cell, which makes an-tibodies.

BACTERIA: organisms that exist on all our body surfaces and in various parts of the body such as the gastrointestinal tract.

BLOCKING ANTIBODY: antibodies found in the pregnant female that block the rejection of the fetus.

BONE MARROW: where the blood cells—white cells, B cells, red cells, and platelets are made.

BUTTERFLY RASH: a butterfly-shaped rash that appears over the bridge of the nose that can be associated with (but not diagnostic of) many diseases, from rosacea to lupus.

CALCIUM CHANNEL BLOCKERS: drugs that act to lower blood pressure by blocking the entry of calcium into cells.

CELL-MEDIATED IMMUNITY: an adaptive immune response in which T cells have the major role.

CHEMOKINES: molecules that stimulate the activation and migration of cells, especially cells that destroy antigens and lymphocytes. They have a central role in the inflammatory process.

CHIMERIC CELL: a cell consisting of two different genetic parts—one half from "self" combined with one half from someone else.

CHOREA: spontaneous movements of the extremities that can occur when an antibody reacts with a part of the brain.

CHRONIC DISEASE: one that lasts for a long time.

CHRONIC FATIGUE SYNDROME: a form of exhaustion, often associated with immune diseases, for which there is no cure or identifiable cause.

CLONE: a population of cells derived from one cell called a progenitor.

COAGULATION: the congealing of blood or the formation of a clot, caused by a cascade of proteins.

COMPLEMENT: a series of proteins that act together to amplify the immune system's attack on foreign antigens.

CORTICOSTEROIDS: steroids naturally derived from the adrenal glands that are part of the "fight or flight" mechanism. They are also manufactured synthetically as the drugs prednisone, cortisone, and dexamethasone.

CORTISONE: one of the many steroids that are used to suppress the immune system. They are produced by the adrenal gland but are also manufactured.

CROSS-REACTION: a situation in which an antibody reacts against a type of tissue that it mistakes for another, that is, the binding of an antibody to an antigen that was not originally the antigen that elicited the antibody.

CRYOGLOBULINEMIA: the presence in the blood of abnormal proteins called cryoglobulins that, in the laboratory, precipitate from blood serum when the temperature is lowered.

CYCLOPHOSPHAMIDE: a very potent immunosuppressive drug that acts by killing rapidly dividing cells.

CYCLOSPORINE A: a potent drug that inhibits communication between T cells.

CYTOKINE: the communication molecules within the immune system, also known as interleukins. These chemicals affect the behavior of cells.

DANOCRINE: a weak male hormone that can raise the number of platelets in the blood.

DEMYELINATION: the removal of the covering (myelin) of the nerve, caused by multiple sclerosis.

DENDRITIC CELLS: cells found in the T-cell areas of the lymph tissues that can be found in various areas of the body such as the skin. These are one form of antigen, presenting cell.

DERMATOMYOSITIS: an inflammatory muscle disease that comes from autoimmunity. It is similar to polymyositis, except that it is associated with a rash.

DHEA (DEHYROEPIANDROSTERONE): a weak androgen that may be used to treat mild forms of diseases such as lupus.

DMARD: acronym for disease-modifying arthritis-related drugs, which are designed to treat the disease process, rather than symptoms.

DNA (DEOXYRIBONUCLEIC ACID): the building blocks of genes. DNA is found in every cell of the body.

ECTODERM: the embryonic group of cells that eventually form the skin, nails, and hair.

EHRLICHIOSIS: a disease that can infect humans as a result of a tick bite. The infection is serious and can be confused with many other diseases such as Lyme disease.

EMBOLUS: a blood clot that travels through the bloodstream.

ENBREL: a surrogate receptor for tumor necrosis factor used to treat many rheumatic diseases, such as rheumatoid arthritis.

ENDORPHINS: natural chemicals that control pain in the human body.

ENDOTHELIUM: the inner lining of the blood vessels.

ERYTHEMA MARGINATUM: the reddish rash found in Lyme disease.

ERYTHROCYTE SEDIMENTATION RATE (ESR): A measure of the degree of inflammation in patients. It is useful in following the effects of therapy with anti-inflammatory drugs.

FIBROMYALGIA: a chronic disorder that causes pain and stiffness throughout tissues that support and move the bones and joints.

FLARE: a period in which disease symptoms reappear or become worse.

GAMMA GLOBULINS: a major class of proteins of which antibodies are a part. Also called immunoglobulins.

GENETIC MARKER: a specific tissue type of gene, similar to a blood type that is passed on from parents to their children.

GRAFT-VERSUS-HOST (GVH): a rejection of tissue that comes from another human that might differ in some genetic way. The immune consequence of such a reaction can result in a disease in some people.

GRAVES' DISEASE: an autoimmune disease in which there is usually overactivity of thyroid function.

HASHIMOTO'S THYROIDITIS: another form of autoimmune thyroid disease. This autoimmune disease of the thyroid can produce underactive thyroid disease in most instances and rarely an overactive thyroid.

HEPATITIS: inflammation of the liver as a result of an immune reaction, a drug, or a virus.

HISTOCOMPATIBILITY: this is the basis for the genetic aspects of the immune system. The ability of one immune system to get along with another.

HLA: the acronym for human leukocyte antigen. This is also known as mixed histocompatibility complex, or the MHC. When the cells of an individual are typed for compatibility before procedures such as a transplant, the HLA markers are measured.

HORROR AUTOTOXICUS: a term meaning "fear of self-poisoning," coined by Paul Ehrlich, one of the early pioneers in immunology. He used it to define the phenomenon that could occur when a person's own defenses turned against him or her—such as what happens in an autoimmune response.

HUMIRA: a monoclonal antibody against the tumor necrosis factor, also called adalimumab.

HYDROXYCHLOROQUINE: an antimalarial drug used to treat autoimmune disease.

HYPERGAMMAGLOBULINEMIA: too much antibody which is the result of an overactive immune system.

HYPOGAMMAGLOBULINEMIA: an immunodeficiency that results from a *depletion* or lack of one or more of the five types of antibody.

IDIOPATHIC THROMBOCYTOPENIC PURPURA (ITP): a disease that causes bleeding and results from the immune destruction of platelets.

IMMUNE RESPONSE: the reaction of the immune system against foreign substances. When this occurs against substances or tissue within the body, it is called an autoimmune reaction.

IMMUNE SYSTEM: a complex system that normally protects the body from infections.

IMMUNODEFICIENCY: the deficiency of cells or antibodies within the immune system that can be mild or life-threatening depending on the missing component.

IMMUNOGENETICS: the inherited part of the immune system. Most of the immunogenetic genes are located on chromosome 6.

IMMUNOGLOBULIN: the scientific name for antibody. There are five major types of immunoglobulins in the blood.

IMURAN: an immunosuppressive drug known as azathioprine.

INFLAMMATION: a local accumulation of fluid, cells, and proteins that arise after an infection, physical injury, or as a result of a local immune response.

INNATE IMMUNITY: the part of the immune system upon which we all depend for the integrity and protection of our body. Innate resistance mechanisms recognize and respond to the presence of certain infectious agents.

INTERLEUKIN: another name for cytokines or communication molecules between cells. They are produced by leukocytes, or white cells.

JOINT: a junction where two bones meet. Most are composed of cartilage, fibrous capsule, synovium, and ligaments.

KETOACIDOSIS: a condition that causes acidification of the blood and is usually the result of fasting, insulin deficiency, or diabetes.

KILLER CELLS: a group of lymphocytes that have antiviral and antitumor activity.

LE CELLS: lupus erythematosus cells that in the past were used to diagnose autoimmune diseases.

LEUKOCYTE: a white cell. These include polymorphonuclear leukocytes (phagocytes), monocytes, and lymphocytes.

LEUKOPHERESIS: removal of cells from the blood of an individual and reinfusion of the liquid portion of the blood.

LUPUS ANTICOAGULANT: an antibody that is directed against an unknown antigen, causing clotting of blood.

LYME DISEASE: an arthritic disease that is not autoimmune in the classic sense. It is caused by the bite of a specific tick, formerly residing on a deer. The immune response to the spirochetes that come from the tick may evolve into an autoimmune form of disease, but it is too early to tell.

LYMPH NODE: these small, bean-shaped centers of activity are strategically placed along the course of the body's lymphatic vessels. They are the seat of immune activity—where the adaptive immune responses originate.

LYMPHOCYTE: cells of the immune system that contain receptors for antigen. There are two kinds of lymphocytes: B cells (humoral immunity) and T cells (cell-mediated immunity).

LYMPHOKINE: a cytokine that is produced by lymphocytes.

MACROPHAGES: one of the cells that attack foreign substances. They also act in the inflammation process and prepare antigens for recognition by other cells.

MAJOR HISTOCOMPATIBILITY COMPLEX (MHC): another name for the immunity genes found on chromosome 6. The MHC is involved in the presentation of antigens to the T cells of the immune system so that they can be recognized.

MENDELIAN: the traditional genetic inheritance as described by the monk Gregor Mendel. It is the one gene-one reaction principle.

MIMICRY: when one molecule is confused for another that is closely related to it in structure.

MRI (MAGNETIC RESONANCE IMAGING): a diagnostic method that uses a magnetic field to examine tissues in great detail.

MRA: magnetic resonance angiography. Uses a magnetic field to examine the flow of blood.

MULTIPLE SCLEROSIS: a central nervous system disease where the insulation of the nerves (myelin) is immunologically attacked and removed. This results in a severe disease that has multiple clinical presentations.

MYCOPHENOLATE: a derivative of a mold that is a part of the anti-rejection drug called CellCept.

MYELIN: a protein that covers some nerves in the brain and the periphery of the body. These nerve covers both insulate nerves and organize them.

MYOPATHIES: inflammatory and noninflammatory diseases of muscle.

MYOSITIS: inflammation of a muscle.

NATURAL KILLER CELLS: another name for killer cells.

NECROSIS: the death of cells due to an immune response injury or because of a chemical such as a drug. This is not the same as apoptosis, or programmed cell death.

NEUTROPHILS: white cells that cause inflammation and carry away cellular debris.

OLIGOCLONAL BANDS: antibody of one type made in the brain and found in the cerebrospinal fluid that helps diagnose multiple sclerosis.

OPTIC NEURITIS: inflammation of the nerves of the eye that can come from many causes, most commonly multiple sclerosis.

PALINDROMIC RHEUMATISM: a form of rheumatoid arthritis in which the symptoms come and go quickly.

PANCREATITIS: inflammation of the pancreas, the organ that produces insulin and helps digest the food.

PANDAS: acronym for pediatric autoimmune neuropsychiatric disease.

PARESTHESIAS: numbness and tingling of the peripheral nerves.

PARVOVIRUS: a virus that can cause a form of anemia or a disease identical to rheumatoid arthritis. It is also the cause of "fifth's" disease (also called slapped cheek syndrome) in children.

PERIARTICULAR OSTEOPENIA: the loss of bone around joints that is most commonly found in early rheumatoid arthritis.

PHAGOCYTOSIS: the process by which cells ingest foreign materials. The ingesting cells are called polymorphonuclear leukocytes.

PHENYLBUTAZONE: a strong anti-inflammatory drug.

PLASMA: the cell-free portion of the blood. Plasma is usually clear.

PLASMA CELLS: matured B cells that are the main family of antibody-secreting cells of the body.

PLASMAPHERESIS: a process that removes plasma from the circulation and then spins out the antibodies. Ultimately, the antibody-free cells are returned to the donor.

PLATELETS: particles derived from cells that are involved in the formation of blood clots. Their absence causes excessive bleeding.

PNEUMOCYSTIS CARINII: a parasite thought to be present in many normal lungs that is often activated in patients with immunodeficiency.

POLYCLONAL ACTIVATION: When the immune system goes on full alert because of a perceived terrorist threat or breach of immune security.

POLYDIPSIA: insatiable thirst.

POLYMYOSITIS: an autoimmune disease of muscle. This is a condition wherein the antibodies are directed toward muscle fibers. It results in pain in and dysfunction of the muscles.

POLYPHAGIA: insatiable appetite.

POLYURIA: frequent urination.

PREDNISONE: a form of cortisone commonly used to treat autoimmune disease. It is the classical immunosuppressant.

PRIMARY BILIARY CIRRHOSIS: a form of autoimmune liver disease that causes cirrhosis.

PROLACTIN: a hormone from the pituitary gland that makes milk appear in the human breast. It can be the result of normal pregnancy or the result of a small tumor.

PROSTAGLANDINS: like leukotrienes, these fatty molecules are derived from arachidonic acid. These potent inflammatory mediators are the targets of the nonsteroidal anti-inflammatory drugs.

PSYCHONEUROIMMUNOLOGY: the new science of the study of the brain-nervous system's interaction with the immune system.

PULMONARY FIBROSIS: thickening of the lining of the lung from a variety of causes, most of which are immune. It often is associated with treatable inflammation, but often is irreversible.

PURPURA: bleeding into the skin as a result of a low level of platelets, clotting factors, or another condition. The results are small, red dots just under the skin.

PUS: thick white material composed of dead cells present in wounds infected with bacteria.

RAYNAUD'S PHENOMENON: a circulatory condition in which the blood vessels in the fingers of the hand are constricted, particularly in cold weather, causing pain and discoloration.

REACTIVE OXYGEN INTERMEDIATES: oxygen atoms that are thought to be a component of the inflammatory process.

RELAXIN: a natural hormone that relaxes the womb during delivery of a baby. It is also thought to have some use in the early stages of scleroderma.

REMICADE: a monoclonal antibody against tumor necrosis factor and used to treat both rheumatoid arthritis and inflammatory bowel disease.

REMISSION: a period when symptoms of disease are reduced (partial remission) or go away completely (complete remission).

RHEUMATIC FEVER: an autoimmune disease that sometimes follows infection with streptococcal organisms. A cross-reacting antibody develops because of the infection, and it can react with multiple tissues and cause significant disease.

RHEUMATOID ARTHRITIS: the most common autoimmune disease; involves inflamed joints and tissues.

RHEUMATOID FACTOR: an anti-antibody that is present in about 60 percent of patients with rheumatoid arthritis. Its strength in the blood does not correlate with disease activity.

RNA (RIBONUCLEIC ACID): a nucleic acid molecule similar to DNA. RNA plays a crucial role in protein synthesis and other cell activities.

SCLERODERMA: an autoimmune disease in which the skin or other organs become laden with collagen.

SEROLOGY: the use of antibodies to measure the presence of antigens in blood. These studies are carried out with clotted blood or serum, not plasma.

SICCA SYNDROME: dry eyes and mouth.

SJÖGREN'S SYNDROME: a disease characterized by the formation of antibody against glands in the body, such as the parotid (saliva-producing) glands and the lachrymal tear-producing glands.

SPIROCHETE: a kind of bacterium. Two well-known spirochetes are those that cause syphilis and Lyme disease.

SUPPRESSOR CELLS: cells that inhibit T-cell responses.

SYMPATHETIC: a part of the nervous system responsible for spontaneous activity such as sweating.

SYSTEMIC LUPUS ERYTHEMATOSUS (ALSO KNOWN AS LUPUS): a condition of chronic inflammation that can cause disease of the skin, heart, lungs, kidneys, joints, and nervous system. When only the skin is involved, the condition is called discoid lupus. When internal organs are involved, the condition is known as systemic lupus erythematosus (SLE).

T CELLS: the key cells in the immune system. These are the targets of antigen presentation and responsible for immunological memory.

T-CELL RECEPTOR: component of the immune cell that helps to recognize an antigen or foreign substance.

TGF: T-cell growth factor, a cytokine.

THROMBOCYTOPENIA: a treatable condition resulting from low blood platelets.

THROMBUS: a stationary blood clot.

THYMUS: an organ that is the site of T-cell development. It sits behind the breastbone, but shrinks away by one's early twenties.

TOLERANCE: the process of desensitizing the immune system. It is the failure of the immune system to react with an antigen, either naturally or by design.

TSH: Thyroid-stimulating hormone. One of the many hormones that come from the pituitary and direct the function of a gland—in this case the thyroid.

TUMOR NECROSIS FACTOR: a major cytokine involved in inflammation. Rheumatoid arthritis and Crohn's disease are treated by lowering its level.

SUGGESTED READING

▷ **Alternative Remedies and Autoimmunity**

J. Horstman, *The Arthritis Foundation's Guide to Alterative Therapies* (Atlanta, GA: The Arthritis Foundation Press, 1999).

> I contributed to the factual nature of this excellent book from the Arthritis Foundation. This book is guaranteed to satisfy your interests in the alternative therapies. Facts are given alongside popular beliefs. I found it to be an excellent guide.

R. Panush, ed., *The Bulletin of the Rheumatic Diseases* (Atlanta, GA: The American College of Rheumatology, 2002).

> This is a summary document for doctors. It is interesting to see the physician's view of alternative therapies.

R. Panush, ed., "Complementary and Alternative Therapies for Rheumatic Disease." In *Rheumatic Diseases of North America* (Philadelphia: W. B. Saunders Company, 1999).

R. Panush, ed., "Complementary and Alternative Therapies for Rheumatic Disease II." In *Rheumatic Diseases of North America* (Philadelphia: W. B. Saunders Company, 2000).

> These are by far the most authoritative text for physicians. They are too complicated for anyone but the most dedicated and fanatical patient. You might require a few years of medical school to read these books, but they do give the most up-to-date information.

▷ **Autoimmune Alopecia**

W. Thompson, J. Shapiro, V. H. Price. *Alopecia Areata: Understanding and Coping with Hair Loss* (Baltimore, MD: Johns Hopkins University Press, 2000).

> Dealing with more than the autoimmune reasons for hair loss, this is a book for patients in particular. There is really nothing I have seen that is available for patients and very little for doctors on this topic. Even the research literature on alopecia seems arcane. This is your best bet.

▷ **Autoimmune Diabetes**

H. P. Chase, *Understanding Insulin-Dependent Diabetes.* (Denver, CO: Children's Diabetes Foundation, 2000).

> Written by a pediatrician, this book is understandable by virtually everyone, although it can be rough going in some areas. The reader will come away with a complete understanding of this illness.

▷ **Drugs Used for the Autoimmune Diseases**

R. G. Lahita, ed., N. Chiorazzi and W. Reeves, assoc. eds., *The Textbook of the Autoimmune Diseases* (Hagerstown, MD: Lippincott Raven Williams and Wilkins, 2001).

> There is no comprehensive text on the treatment of the autoimmune diseases. Some of the books I have recommended above will deal with treatment, but new and innovative methods of treating these diseases will come either from a textbook, from the web, or from the various organizations that are listed as agencies that deal with the autoimmune diseases.

▷ **General Autoimmunity**

R. G. Lahita, ed., N. Chiorazzi and W. Reeves, assoc. ed., *The Textbook of the Autoimmune Diseases.* (Hagerstown, MD: Lippincott Raven Williams and Wilkins, 2001).

> This authoritative textbook is geared to the professional. It deals with all aspects of autoimmune disease, including many topics not covered in this book. Seventy-nine authors cover every topic and disease that involves autoimmunity.

Suggested Reading

▷ **Low Platelets**

T. S. Kickler and J. H. Herman, eds., *Current Issues in Platelet Transfusion Therapy and Platelet Alloimmunity* (Bethesda, MD: American Association of Blood Banks, 2002).

> This book is really for professionals. However, those with a burning desire to learn about platelets and problems associated with them could read this book and might learn something.

▷ **Multiple Sclerosis**

D. Barnes and I. McDonald, *Multiple Sclerosis: Questions and Answers* (West Palm Beach, FL: Merit Publishing International, 2000).

> This book is primarily aimed at doctors, but can be of interest to patients and caregivers who want the latest information on MS.

J. L. Nichols, *Women Living with Multiple Sclerosis* (Alameda, CA: Hunter House, 1999).

> Written by a patient, this book is excellent for others suffering from common care and quality-of-life issues.

▷ **Mystery Diseases (Fibromyalgia and Silicone Implants)**

C. Cunningham, *The Fibromyalgia Relief Handbook* (Encinitas, CA: United Research Publishing. 2000).

> Patients swear that this book makes them better. It deals with alternative solutions to pain in a rather difficult and medically confusing disease.

S. Bondurant and V. L. Ernster, eds., *Safety of Silicone Breast Implants*

> This is a book for clinicians and researchers. The entire issue of silicone implants is thorny, and this book deals with the data in a fair way. New York: National Academy Press, 2000.

▷ **Other Enigmas of Autoimmunity**

R. G. Lahita, ed., N. Chiorazzi and W. Reeves, assoc. eds., *The Textbook of the Autoimmune Diseases* (Hagerstown, MD: Lippincott Raven Williams and Wilkins, 2001).

> This is the only detailed book I know of that deals with the enigmas of autoimmunity.

Suggested Reading

▷ **Rheumatoid Arthritis**

R. G. Lahita, *Rheumatoid Arthritis: Everything You Need to Know* (New York: Avery Press, 2001).
> Written for patients in question-and-answer format. This is a good introduction to the disease.

The Arthritis Foundation, *Rheumatoid Arthritis* (Atlanta: The Arthritis Foundation, 2001).
> This is an excellent reference pamphlet for patients.

R. Panush et al., ed., *The Yearbook of Rheumatology, Arthritis and Musculoskeletal Disease* (St. Louis: Mosby Books, published yearly).
> This series is meant to highlight articles of great interest each year in the field of rheumatology and autoimmunity. The commentaries are candid and written by an expert. This is primarily for physicians.

▷ **Scleroderma**

M. D. Mayes, *The Scleroderma Book: A Guide for Patients and Families* (New York: Oxford University Press, 1999).
> A good book to get a handle on a very serious and confusing illness.

▷ **Sjögren's Syndrome**

Elaine Harris, ed., *The Sjögren's Syndrome Handbook* (Bethesda, MD: Sjögren's Syndrome Foundation, 1989).
> This book is written for patients and is a good reference work for the disease.

▷ **Streptococcal Infection and Psychiatry**

R. R. Trifiletti and A. M., Packard "Immune Mechanisms in Pediatric Neuropsychiatric Disorders: Tourette's Syndrome, OCD and PANDAS," *Child Adolescent Psychiatric Clinics of North America* 8(4), 767–775 (1999).
> A scientific paper that deals with the issues of immune mechanisms and pediatric disease.

Suggested Reading

▷ Systemic Lupus Erythematosus

R. G. Lahita, *What Is Lupus?* (Rockville, MD: Lupus Foundation of America Publications, 2001).

> This is the standard pamphlet for people newly diagnosed with the disease. It can be found free online at the Lupus Foundation website. It is also available in bulk for a modest fee.

Arthritis Foundation, *The Lupus Pamphlet* (Atlanta: Arthritis Foundation, 2002).

> This pamphlet is also very informative and written for the lay person.

R. G. Lahita and R. H. Phillips, *Lupus: Q&A* (New York: Avery Publishing, 2004).

> A book written for the patient. The information is given in question and answer format.

Daniel Wallace, *The Lupus Book* (New York: Oxford Press, 1995).

> Another book written for the patient by an acknowledged expert. It is quite excellent.

R. G. Lahita, *Systemic Lupus Erythematosus*, 3rd ed. (San Diego: Academic Press: 1999).

> A book for the professional. This reference work includes forty-nine contributors on all aspects of the disease.

▷ The Antiphospholipid Syndrome

R. G. Lahita, *Systemic Lupus Erythematosus*, 3rd ed. (San Diego: Academic Press, 1999).

> This book has an entire section dedicated to antiphospholipid syndrome.

G. V. H. Hughes, *The Hughes Syndrome, A Patient's Guide*, 1st ed. (New York: Springer Verlag, 2001).

> Dr. Hughes, considered by many to be the discoverer of this disease, has written a wonderful book to explain this syndrome to laypeople.

Suggested Reading

M. Khamashta, ed., *The Hughes Syndrome* (London: Elsevier Press, 2001).

> A compendium of papers on this important disease written by Dr. Hughes's friends and colleagues. This is for the professional.

Ronald Asherson, ed., *The Antiphospholipid Syndrome* (London: Elsevier Press, 2002).

> The textbook for this illness, edited for the professional.

▷ The Immune System

C. Janeway, P. Travers, M. Walport, and M. Shlomchik, *Immunobiology*, 5th ed. (New York: Garland Publications, 2001).

> This is the book that I use to teach medical residents and young physicians about basic immunology. It is a bit complicated but will be worth it for the very enthusiastic reader. The figures are terrific.

▷ Vasculitis and the Circulation

E. Ball and S. Louis Bridges Jr., eds., *Vasculitis* (New York: Oxford University Press, 2001).

> This is a comprehensive review of this very difficult topic. Issues of diagnosis, treatment, and pathogenesis of the disease are discussed. May be a bit heavy for the average reader.

HELPFUL ORGANIZATIONS

**American Autoimmune Related
   Diseases Association**
22100 Gratiot Avenue
East Detroit, MI 48021-2227
1-586-776-3900
www.aarda.org

American Diabetes Association
1701 North Beauregard Street
Alexandria, VA 22311
1-800-Diabetes
www.diabetes.org

American Liver Foundation
Greater New York Chapter
50 Broadway
New York, NY 10004
1-877-307-7507
www.liverfoundation.org

American Thyroid Association
6066 Leesburg Pike, Suite 650
Falls Church, VA 22041
1-800-thyroid
www.thyroid.org

Arthritis Foundation
National Office
PO Box 7669
Atlanta, GA 30357-0669
1-800-283-7800
www.arthritis.org

**Juvenile Diabetes Foundation
   International**
120 Wall Street
New York, NY 10005-4001
1-800-533-CURE
www.jdf.org

Lupus Foundation of America
2000 L Street, NW, Suite 710
Washington, DC 20036
1-202-349-1155
www.lupus.org

Myositis Association of America
1233 20th Street NW, Suite 402
Washington, DC 20036
1-202-887-0088
www.myositis.org

**National Alopecia Areata
  Foundation**
PO Box 150760
San Rafael, CA 94915-0760
1-415-472-3780
www.naaf.org

National Multiple Sclerosis Society
733 Third Avenue, 6th floor
New York, NY 10017-3288
1-800-Fight MS
www.nationalmssociety.org

**National Organization for Rare
  Disorders**
55 Kenosia Avenue
PO Box 1968
Danbury, CT 06813-1968
1-203-744-0100
www.rarediseases.org

Sjögren's Syndrome Foundation
8120 Woodmont Avenue
Bethesda, MD 20814
1-301-718-0300
www.sjogrens.com

The SLE Foundation
149 Madison Avenue, Suite 205
New York, NY 10016
1-212-685-4118
www.lupusny.org

United Scleroderma Foundation
89 Newberry Street, Suite 201
Danvers, MA 01923
1-800-722-4673
www.scleroderma.org

INDEX

Index

anakinra, 227, 229
analgesics, 98, 206
androgens, 6, 14, 23, 31
anemia, 122, 133, 225
angiogenesis factor, 139
ankylosing spondylitis, 228
anlage, 134
anorexia, 95
antibiotics, 28, 94, 106, 254
  for rheumatic fever, 101–2, 103
  for vasculitis, 113, 114
antibodies, xv, 5, 163
  anti-brain-nucleus, 91, 95
  antiphospholipid syndrome and,
    40–44, 46, 47–48, 127
  defined, 4
  diabetes and, 65, 66
  idiopathic thrombocytopenic purpura
    and, 54, 59
  intravenous, 94, 231
  liver disease and, 166
  in long-term vs. short-term immunity,
    9
  lupus and, 119, 121, 125–26, 130,
    254–55
  mimicry and, 18
  muscle disease and, 184–85
  PANDAS and, 90, 91, 92, 94, 95
  plasma cells and, 8
  pooled, 59
  rheumatoid arthritis and, 148, 150,
    198
  rheumatoid factor and, 194–95
  scleroderma and, 178
  silicone implant syndrome and, 210,
    211
  Sjögren's syndrome and, 146, 147,
    148, 150, 153
  therapeutic, 33
  thyroid disease and, 156–59
  vasculitis and, 108, 111–12, 113
anticardiolipin, 47, 48
anticoagulants, 39, 45, 49
antidepressants, 114, 206

anti-DNA antibodies, 126
antigen exposure theory, 28
antigens, 4–9, 48, 54, 59, 163
  B cells and, 8, 9
  defined, 4
  diabetes and, 66
  external, 4, 8–9, 18, 19
  immune memory and, 8–9
  internal, 4–5, 19
  lupus and, 121
  mimicry and, 18
  multiple sclerosis and, 86–87
  muscle disease and, 184–85
  T cells and, 6–7, 9, 76
  thyroid disease and, 156
  tolerance and, 233
anti-inflammatory drugs, 98, 99, 101,
  151, 188, 246
  for lupus, 126–27
  nonsteroidal (NSAID), 126–27,
    199–200, 217–20
anti-LA antibody, 150
antimalarial drugs, 127, 128, 137, 138,
  222–23, 226
antineutrophilic cytoplasmic antibody
  (ANCA), 112
antinuclear antibodies (ANA), 110–11,
  125–26, 150, 187, 194
antiphospholipid (sticky blood)
  syndrome (APLS), xiv–xv, 27,
  37–50, 81, 252
  causes of, 41, 103
  defined, 40–41
  diagnosis of, 45–48
  lupus and, 40, 42, 122, 124, 127
  multiple miscarriage and, 26, 42,
    44–45
  symptoms of, 37–40
  three components of, 41–45
  thrombocytopenia and, 42, 43–44
  thrombosis and, 40, 42–43, 46, 47
  treatment of, 48–50
anti-RO antibody, 146, 150, 153
anti-Smith antigen, 126

Index

Index

Index

Index

Index